OFFICIALLY
DISCARDED
PILATES AND PREGNANCY

A workbook for before, during and after pregnancy

Sarah Picot

Forewords by James Powers, M.D. and Francis Bergin jr., M.D. OB/GYNs

Collin Cullen, M.D.

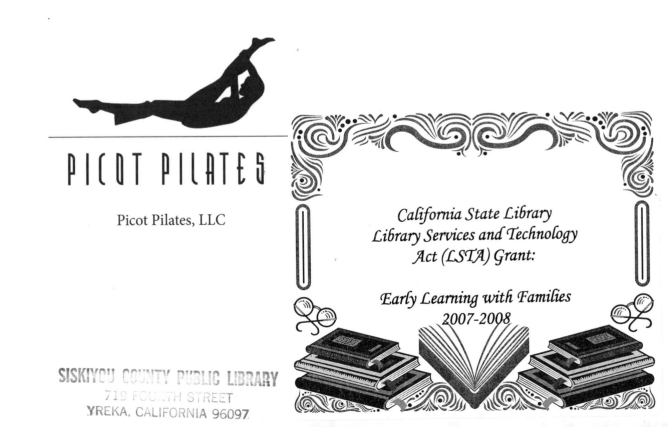

PICOT PILATES

Picot Pilates, LLC

*California State Library
Library Services and Technology
Act (LSTA) Grant:*

*Early Learning with Families
2007-2008*

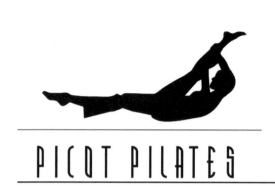

PICOT PILATES

Pilates and Pregnancy. Copyright © 2006 by Sarah Picot.

Edited by Amy Friedlander

Illustrated by Todd Gardner

Design and layout by Jim Beals

Visit www.picotpilates.com for more information.

Pilates and Pregnancy: A workbook for before, during and after pregnancy/by Sarah Picot. – 2nd ed.

ISBN: 0-9778150-1-3

Library of Congress Control Number: 2006906819

Disclaimer: The ideas and suggestions in this book are not meant to be construed as medical advice. Seek permission from your doctor before starting this or any other exercise program. This program is not meant to be used by women who have a history of miscarriage, pre-eclampsia, bleeding, or incompetent cervix, or who are are carrying multiples.

Dedication:

For my husband Steve and beautiful sons Stevie and Ben for their support, patience and inspiration.

I would also like to dedicate this book to my mother for her unending belief in me. She has always made it possible for me to follow my dreams.

Acknowledgements

I would like to thank:

Drs. Francis T. Bergin, Collin Cullen and James Powers for their time, wisdom and support.

Laura Edmiston, Sheri Walczy and midwife/instructor Dominique Galante for their professional contributions to the birth of the Prenatal Pilates and Post-natal Pilates video series.

Dana Dowd, Kristine Bishop and Margo M. Sadow for being such beautiful models for this book.

Master teacher Gina Papallia for giving me my love of Pilates.

Amy Friedlander for editing this book with such skill and adding her own appreciation and knowledge of The Method to this project.

Todd Gardner for his creative gift of graphic design.

Jim Beals for his attention to detail in laying out this book.

For all the past, present and future Pilates practitioners who appreciate the brilliance of the Joseph Pilates Method and keep his Method alive and growing.

Foreword

It is apparent that a comprehensive prenatal exercise program does help to promote flexibility, relaxation, strength and confidence to handle pregnancy and its debilitating body changes and to promote an easier labor experience in the relatively difficult and demanding second stage of labor.

The videotape based on the "Pilates" exercise program is well designed and offers gentle, gradual muscle strengthening and flexibility training that, in our experience, aids greatly in toning muscle groups during all trimesters. In addition, it promotes effective relaxation during labor and strength training for pushing during that phase of expulsion of the newborn.

We believe that a strict adherence to these well designed Pilates exercises will enhance every pregnant mother's antepartum care for nine months and will shorten labor and delivery for those mothers who take time to participate faithfully in these programs.

Great credit should be given to the author for her dedication and patience in explaining in detail the exercises and demonstrating that they did, in fact, work in her own labor.

This prenatal exercise program is a welcome addition to the already crowded field of childbirth preparation myths, but one which we believe will be of great use to the countless mothers who will undoubtedly find it a godsend in their quest for "natural" childbirth.

Dr. James S. Powers *OB/GYN*
Dr. Francis T. Bergin *OB/GYN*
Fellows of the American College of OB/GYN
Both rated among the top doctors in the Washington area
  in 1999 according to the Washingtonian Magazine

2002

Pilates and Pregnancy

Section II: Machine Exercises

Section III: The Postnatal Workout

Introduction

Hi, my name is Sarah Picot. I am a certified Pilates instructor, dance teacher and mother of two boys.

If you are reading this book, congratulations are in order! Either you've decided to prepare your body for pregnancy, or you are pregnant. You may even have given birth to your baby. Like me, you want to make your pregnancy and labor more comfortable, shorten your delivery and re-shape your postnatal body.

I was dancing professionally in New York City and training at Tribecca Body Works and The Pilates Studio to become a Pilates instructor when I became pregnant with my first son. I wanted to continue to work out because I knew the benefits to my endurance, strength and posture would be great. However, I was apprehensive about safety.

I soon discovered a dearth of resources. I asked everyone for advice, including master teachers. But no one had concrete answers for me. I was told I could continue to do Pilates throughout my pregnancy by modifying here and there. In the same breath, I was told I would not be allowed to continue with The Pilates Studio's certification program at that time because they felt it would become too difficult later in my pregnancy.

So, what did it mean to "modify" the program? What would be safe? I had enough kinesthetic knowledge to know that notions of safety would change as my body changed. For example, one suggestion was to do **ROLL-UP**—an exercise that sort of resembles a sit-up with straight legs. That would be fine during the first trimester. But I knew that even with a modification that would bend my knees to relieve some of the strain on my back, there was no way I could or should try the exercise during my last trimester. So I ended up in prenatal yoga classes, of which there are many. The yoga world realizes the importance of providing specifically designed modifications for a pregnant woman. But good as yoga is, I still hankered for the benefits of Pilates, even while pregnant.

I was still pregnant when my husband Steve and I moved to Washington. After our first son Stevie was born, I finished getting my certification through the PhysicalMind Institute. Since I was a brand-new mother, I found clients and other instructors coming to me for advice on practicing Pilates while pregnant. Since most women do not have the fitness and health knowledge to modify the exercises by themselves, any more than I really did when I first became pregnant, I decided to do some research.

You have the results in your hands. After consulting doctors, nurses, physical therapists and other Pilates instructors, I have developed a prenatal Pilates program designed to meet your body's unique requirements in each trimester. I was able to work out and improve upon my prenatal program using my own body because I had become pregnant with my second son just as I had finished my research.

These exercises are designed to be done at home with the help of household items. All you will need are one towel, two soup cans, three firm blankets, two or three pillows and comfortable workout clothes.

Before we get started, let me take a moment to introduce you to Joseph Pilates and then to talk about how the Pilates program of exercise can work your body through your pregnancy and beyond. I believe this program is safe. But throughout, remember to listen to your body. If something doesn't feel right to your body, stop.

Section I: The Program

Who Was Joseph Pilates?

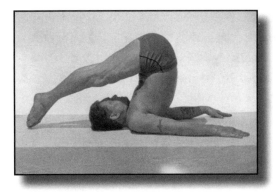

JOSEPH PILATES

PHOTO COURTESY OF THE PILATES METHOD ALLIANCE

Joseph Pilates was born in Germany in 1880. A sickly child, he overcame many physical weaknesses by concentrating on body building, boxing and gymnastics and maintained a lifelong fascination with the power of the human body. After moving to England, he worked at various jobs, including one as a circus performer. World War I broke out in 1914 and he was interned. While in the internment camp, Pilates became a nurse and began training the other internees in his workout routine, a combination of traditional calisthenics tempered with the mind/body meditative connection found in Eastern cultures. It was said that his exercises helped prevent all of his fellow detainees from falling ill from influenza in the epidemic that killed thousands in England in 1918.

After the war ended, Pilates emigrated from Europe to the United States. On the ship coming over, he met his future wife Clara, and they opened a studio in New York City. There, he finetuned his exercises into a method he called "Contrology." Over 500 individual exercises were developed with the emphasis on abdominal strength, serious concentration on the mechanics of the body and stretching. Pilates was a walking advertisement for his method, remaining in incredible health and fitness until his death in a fire in 1967 at the age of 87.

In the years since Pilates died, his students and their students have preserved, interpreted and evolved his work. There are now three principal centers: The Pilates Studio in New York, The Pilates Center in Boulder, and PhysicalMind Institute, also located in New York, where I did some of my training. Dancers and other athletes have sworn by his method. George Balanchine and Martha Graham studied with him and had their dancers do so as well. More recently, celebrities such as Madonna, Courtney Cox-Arquette and Gwyneth Paltrow have helped give Pilates wider exposure. Stars, celebrities, professional performers, athletes, gym rats and novices have all discovered the truth in Pilates' mantra: you will feel better in ten visits, look better in twenty and have a new body in thirty. Stay with it and you will too!

Now, let's get started.

What is Pilates?

So what exactly is **Pilates**? (Pronounced "peh la tees".)

Pilates is an exercise program that incorporates the entire body and mind to achieve length, strength and power with an intense focus on the core. Eastern principles of concentration, conscious breathing and stretching are combined with Western views of calisthenics for strength and endurance. Properly followed, the program improves posture, elongates muscles and flattens the stomach.

Most universal gyms and training programs target one group or a few muscle groups during a single exercise. These programs tend to focus on the largest and most topical muscles, potentially leaving your body disjointed and not working at an optimal level. When one type of muscle is overused, an imbalance occurs, and strains and injuries are the probable results.

Unlike conventional calisthenics, **Pilates** requires a constant awareness of the muscle groups that need to be activated during the different exercises. Most people have no knowledge of how their bodies are built or how and why they move. Ironically, most of us wouldn't expect to get the optimum use out of our computers or cars without a basic understanding of their mechanics. So we educate ourselves with manuals and or classes. To achieve the most from this program, you need to educate yourself and be aware of what muscles you are using and where they are. **Pilates** requires you to include your mind in your workout and think before you move.

Muscles are found in layers. We tend only to use the largest and most external muscles, like the **quadriceps** in the thigh or the **rectus** in the abdomen. **Pilates** asks you to work from the inside out, to find the deeper muscles that support the body. Without this inward seeking process, it would be like building a house with a very strong roof and walls yet leaving the foundation weak. It would be only a matter of time before it would fall apart.

Finding these deep muscles can be very difficult – like learning to wiggle your ears. The big muscles always want to take over. While everyone has the musculature to do it, few have figured out where those muscles are or how to access them. That's where **Pilates** comes in. The program teaches you how to find and strengthen those "hidden" muscles so that you always work from your core, from your "**powerhouse**."

The "**powerhouse**" (Figure 1) is a **Pilates** term that refers to the muscles in the abdomen and back that run from the lower ribcage to the pelvis. They are essential in all movement. The abdominals, for instance, must be toned and actively working to protect the back and control torso movement in every exercise. While one muscle group is being called on to contract, others must work in opposition to lengthen; still others must stabilize the rest of the body. In this way, the body is always working efficiently as a cooperative unit. For example, raising your leg becomes an abdominal, pelvic and thigh exercise.

Muscles are asked to lengthen, rather than compress, before they are activated. The goal is to achieve more space in the body, especially the spine, which increases blood flow and hence mobility. The lengthening of the limbs trains the muscles to stay long. This lengthening coupled with the stability of the "**powerhouse**" produces flexibility. If you tilt your **pelvis** and tuck your **tailbone** under while trying to stretch the back of the leg, you will get a false sense of how flexible your leg is. Keeping the **pelvis** stabile and the **tailbone** connected to the floor, separates it from the torso and allows deep stretching to take place. Strength, length and flexibility—all reasons why dancers have known the value of **Pilates** for years.

Since the work is so deep and intense, **Pilates** requires far fewer repetitions than the calisthenics you probably did in high school

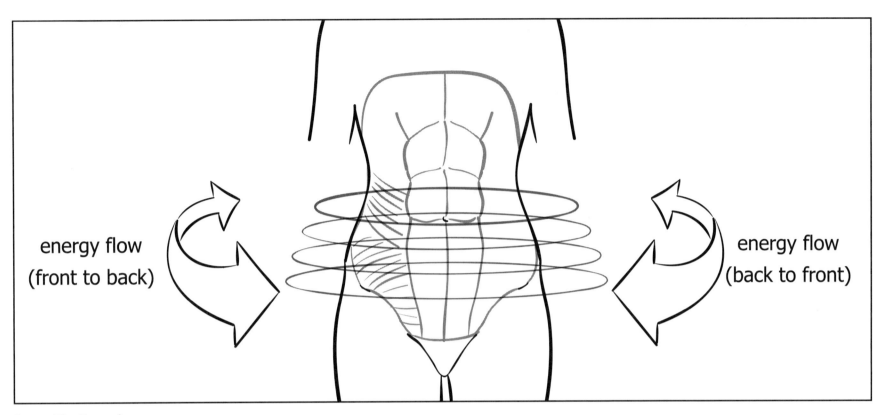

energy flow
(front to back)

energy flow
(back to front)

Figure 1. **The Powerhouse.**

phys ed. **Joseph Pilates** believed that fewer repetitions of specific exercises done well were more valuable than a hundred performed without care. Fifty crunches with your **rectus abdominus** pushed out, your **pelvis** tilted and your shoulders hunched will not leave you stronger than five ROLL UPS done correctly. (Figures 2a & 2b) The emphasis in this Pilates "sit-up" is on pulling in the abdominals, keeping your neck long and your hip flexors relaxed, which will not only leave you with a flatter stomach but also better posture and a healthier back. Now, you ask, how does this work during pregnancy? Keep reading.

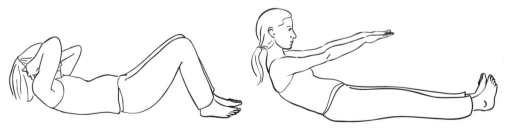

Figure 2a. **Bad crunches**

Figure 2b. **Roll up**

How is Pilates compatible with pregnancy?

Your pregnant body is prone to strains and pulls. The sudden increase in weight puts tremendous pressure on your back, shoulders and legs. Joints loosen in preparation for labor, as the pregnancy hormone **Relaxin** floods your system. Providing nutrients for a growing fetus is an aerobic workout in itself. Your body requires more oxygen and twice the blood volume.

Pilates focuses on gentle movement performed in a safe range of motion, which is essential for your pregnant body. Pregnancy puts enough demands on your body without asking it to accept jarring, straining or stressful movements. The exercises in this book have been carefully adapted to meet the changes, demands and discomforts particular to each stage of pregnancy.

As your baby grows, the weight strains on your back and shoulders help ruin posture, leaving your body susceptible to aches and pains. **Pilates** targets the abdominal region and is always conscious of protecting the back. Training your abdominals to work deeply to support your internal organs and back will make your pregnancy more comfortable. (Figure 3a & 3b)

This deep abdominal work feels similar to doing **Kegels** (See Terms and Techniques.). If you are not already familiar with how to **Kegel**, learn! **Kegels** are crucial for all women to master. They are especially important for pregnant and post-natal women because they help to strengthen the **pelvic floor**, which will contribute to bladder control. **Kegeling** also tightens the vaginal wall, which can get overstretched during a vaginal delivery.

One of the worst things a pregnant woman can do is to sit or stand in one position for too long. The increase in blood and fluid volume along with weight gain contributes to **edema** (swelling) and **varicosities** (varicose veins) in the legs. The act of working the entire body together with the conscious **Pilates breathing technique**, which oxygenates the blood, helps you minimize these problems by improving circulation (like all exercise).

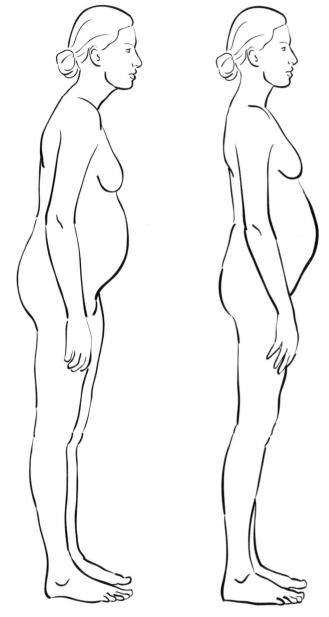

Figure 3a. **Typical pregnancy posture**   Figure 3b. **Correct posture**

Probably the most important benefit of this work for a pregnant woman is the abdominal muscle memory that can be achieved. Muscle memory is your body's ability to reactivate the strength and purpose of a particular muscle automatically. You can improve your body's muscle memory by teaching your muscles where, when and how to activate.

The effort and concentration on body awareness that **Pilates** requires will pay off at the end of your pregnancy. Conscious movement will become, to a large degree, unconscious, much like swallowing or walking. You won't even feel like you have muscles, but they are there. Your body will still work to support you and will have the ability to find the proper muscles for pushing, during labor and delivery.

Most first time mothers and women who have had epidurals tend to have longer pushing times during delivery. They either don't know which muscles to use for pushing and where they are, or they simply can't feel them. Finding those deep muscles over and over again in these exercises trains your brain and body to remember how to activate a given muscle when needed. As your pregnancy progresses, you can expect your stamina and comfort levels to change, too.

As a first trimester mother-to-be, you may feel fatigued and nauseous yet able to lie on

Having had an epidural with both my deliveries, I know the power of muscle memory. Pilates targets the deep, low abdominals used in the pushing phase of labor. I had worked those deep transverse and oblique muscles enough to where it was easy to call them into action even though I couldn't actually feel them. Since Stevie was my first and he hadn't dropped into my pelvis at all, he took a little longer. Just over an hour. But my doctor was amazed that I found the right muscles on my first push. My second son Ben, who was bigger than Stevie, only took ten minutes of pushing. My doctor remarked that my relatively short and easy deliveries made me a walking advertisement for Pilates and pregnancy.

Muscle memory is an amazing thing!

WHAT CAN YOU EXPECT?

First Trimester	Second Trimester	Third Trimester
Fatigue	Relief from morning sickness	Breathlessness
Nausea	More energy	Fatigue
Swollen/tender breasts	Nasal congestion	Backaches
Frequent urination	Hair/skin changes	Clumsiness
Vivid dreams	Feeling warmer	Braxton Hicks contractions*

*Braxton Hicks contractions are preparatory contractions or a tightening of the uterus. They are usually painless and do not occur in regular intervals, the way labor contractions do

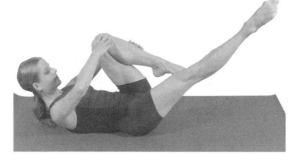

First Trimester

your back for long periods of time. You will be able to work closer to the original exercises and target your deep abdominal muscles. The focus on fewer repetitions will help you not overexert your body. The muscle memory developed during this trimester will be crucial when you are so overstretched later in your pregnancy that you won't even feel like you even have muscles.

In your second trimester, you will probably feel more energetic. This trimester is usually thought of as the "golden time." Most women no longer feel sick or as tired and may want to take advantage of new-found flexibility and energy. Even so, you must be mindful of your body temperature and the **relaxin** in your system or you may be apt to over exert yourself. Limiting movements within the confines of your body will help protect unstable joints. The fact that **Pilates** is not a very aerobic exercise program (unless you are more advanced and able to flow straight through all the exer-

cises without pausing) makes worrying about raising your core temperature less urgent.

After the fourth month, you may not be able to lie on your back as long as you could earlier in your pregnancy because of the weight of your growing uterus on the **vena cava** (Figure 4), the artery which supplies blood to both mother and baby. Even though you may not feel sick lying on your back, some doctors feel blood flow may still be compromised and recommend staying off your back. Propping up on an incline makes the second trimester's exercises more comfortable. The incline and the modifications for this position also begin to shift some of the demand to the legs, buttocks and upper abdominal muscles.

As you enter your third trimester, your internal organs have been pushed high into your thoracic cavity (**ribcage**), making it difficult to breathe (Figure 5). **Pilates'** use of lateral and back **breathing** is a wonderful way to alleviate that discomfort. This **ribcage breathing**

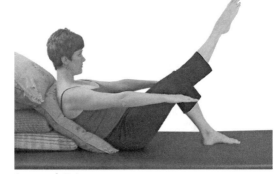

Second Trimester

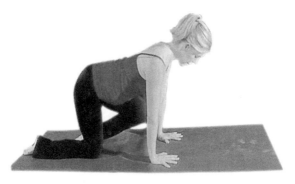

Third Trimester

increases the space between the ribs giving your lungs more room to fill and to fill to greater capacity. You will be able to oxygenate your blood better with each breath.

Retraining your abdomen to remain toned while breathing and allowing your ribs and back to expand also eases the shortness of breath that comes when your **diaphragm** isn't able to drop into the abdomen as deeply as it did before you become pregnant. The deeper and fuller breaths that come from the **Pilates' breathing technique** are very helpful during contractions (See Terms and Techniques.). The increase in lung capacity that develops allows for greater stamina, which will help get you through the many hours of labor.

By twenty-eight weeks, the fatigue is back, and the sheer size of your abdomen makes limiting ranges of motion more necessary. You won't be able to lie on your back for too long because of the pressure the uterus places

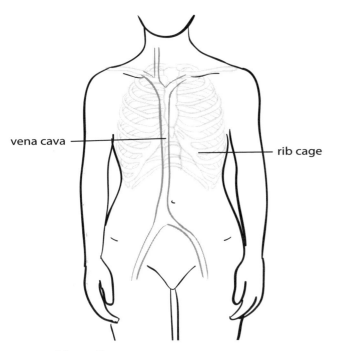

vena cava

rib cage

FIGURE 4. **Vena Cava**

Now, most women find themselves thinking that their flat stomach was sacrificed for motherhood. Not so. This work can bring back a flat or at least flatter stomach like nothing else. Once the deep muscles have been discovered and trained, they tend to return to their pre-pregnancy shape faster. This won't happen on their own, they still need to be exercised and worked in the same fashion. Much like an overstretched rubber band, eventually those muscles can go back to their original shape.

Even the postpartum mom will need some modifications to accommodate soreness and fatigue. The essential question at this point is how to exercise with a baby at your side? By including your baby in the workout. These exercises can be a lot of fun to do with your baby as a participant. She can be placed in a bouncy seat, supportive pillow or on your lap and stomach.

Don't expect miracles. This workout will not do it on its own. Concentration, consistency, a balanced diet and lifestyle and cardiovascular exercises all work together to achieve the healthy prenatal and postnatal body we all want.

on the **vena cave**, which can stop blood flow to both you and the baby. The exercises can be done sitting, kneeling or standing at this stage in the pregnancy as I demonstrate in the third trimester workout.

After the thirty-sixth week of pregnancy, I suggest an exercise blackout. Take advantage of this time to rest and work on your **Pilates Breathing technique**. Of course you may still choose relaxation exercises like CAT or CHILD'S POSE. Delivery is a long process that takes all of your energy. You will have prepared your body very well; now is the time to pamper yourself. It may be hard to wait out the last days, but pretty soon, you will deliver, and after all that hard work, you have a beautiful baby.

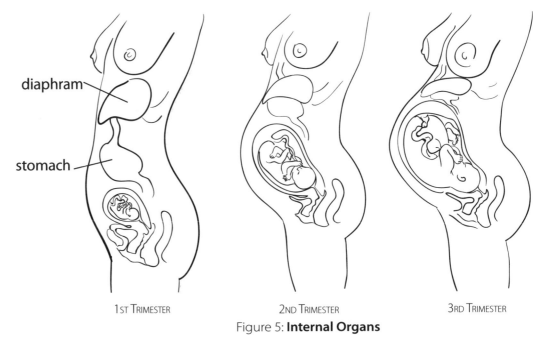

diaphram

stomach

1ST TRIMESTER   2ND TRIMESTER   3RD TRIMESTER

Figure 5: **Internal Organs**

Who and When?

How fit should you be to do this program? The exercises I have chosen are a mix of fundamentals and basic **Pilates** mat exercises that are necessary for everyone. However you will still need to discuss your exercise choices with your doctor to make sure they are right for you. Even the most advanced **Pilates** devotee needs to tone down her workout a bit during her pregnancy. You won't be able to do the more advanced exercises comfortably, safely or, perhaps, correctly. The beauty of **Pilates** is that the most basic movements can give you the most intense workout. Some of the exercises may be too difficult to do in their original format. I have added modifications for almost all of the exercises to make this workout suitable for just about everyone.

How should you take advantage of this book's format so that it benefits your particular fitness level? Rate your pre-pregnancy fitness level from 1 to 5, a 1 being a couch potato and a 5 being a marathon runner. Be honest! If you are closer to a 1, go slowly. Start with just a few basic exercises such as **BREATHING, CAT** and **SPINE STRETCH**, but do them consistently. Add more of the routine as you build your strength and stamina. Pregnancy hormones will drive you deeper into a state of lethargy, so make it part of your daily routine to do at least some light exercise. Remember that something is better than nothing. (Unless you have been placed on bed rest, of course.) See "How to Use This Book" to find the exercises that are right for you.

Ideally you should do something everyday. Try some low impact cardio exercises four times per week and **Pilates** three times a week. Walking and swimming are great complements to this work. Don't be discouraged by the apparent difficulty of an exercise. Do the simplest modification. It is just important that you move.

If you are a level 1, watch your diet. An inactive mother who eats an unhealthy diet is more likely to give birth to an overweight baby and increases her likelihood of developing gestational diabetes and high blood pressure. Don't be fooled by the phrase, "you're eating for two". This refers to quality not quantity.

If you are closer to a 5, don't feel too confident in the healthiness of your normal exercise routine for your baby and your pregnant body. You will have to cut back on the amount of exercise you would normally do. Such a fine-tuned body will tend to be selfish and take nutrients and oxygenated blood away from the fetus in order to keep your well-honed body going at the same level. Very active women tend to have underweight and premature babies. The American Medical Association recommends that very active women do whatever they did before they became pregnant but that they cut their programs in half during the first twenty weeks and then cut that regimen in half for the last twenty weeks.

Obviously, mountain climbing, skiing, skydiving or anything where falls can bring trauma to the baby are unwise activities to continue.

As with any program, consult your doctor before starting. Any woman with a history of miscarriage, incompetent cervix, multiple fetuses, placenta previa, ruptured membranes, preeclampsia, risk of premature labor or bleeding problems should not do this or any other exercise program. In addition, you should stop what ever you are doing and call your doctor if you experience vaginal bleeding, shortness of breath prior to exercising, dizziness, headache, calf pain or swelling, decreased fetal movement or leakage of amniotic fluid.

If you have never done **Pilates** before, please do the easier modification. If the choice, for instance, is between having your legs or your head up and leaving them on the floor, put them down! Not every exercise will be right for every body. If an exercise does not feel right today, skip it. If you have done **Pilates** before—and even if you are advanced—it is better to adhere to the variations in this book. Your pregnant body is not the same as it was, even if it feels like it is. The exercises may feel too easy. They are not. These are geared specifically for the pregnant body. As you get bigger, the same exercises will become more difficult to perform. This isn't a contest. Don't try and prove that you can still do it the advanced way. Morning sickness, fatigue, the hormone **relaxin** and your growing fetus will all require cutting back a bit.

The doctors I have consulted recommend a blackout period from one to seven weeks of pregnancy and after the thirty-sixth week. Fifty percent of all bleeding occurs in the first seven weeks of pregnancy. Even though there is no causal link between exercise and miscarrage during this time it is better to wait for this stessful period to pass. After the thirty-sixth week, you are so close to delivering that you won't have much energy to workout. Continue to do light cardio and get all the rest you can.

Lying on your back anytime after the fourth month may begin to be uncomfortable. By the twenty-eighth week, the weight of the uterus can cut off blood supply to you and your baby. Work-ing on an incline and changing positions during your second trimester and staying off your back completely during your third trimester should help. Regardless, if you begin to feel nauseous or dizzy, roll onto your left side.

After your fourth month intense abdominal activity that focuses on your rectus abdominous should be avoided. Many women experience a separation of that muscle during pregnancy. We don't want to put too much burden on an already overstretched muscle (Figure 6, diastasis).

Morning sickness can put a damper on anyone's motivation. Keep crackers by your side. An empty stomach invites queasiness. Try to eat six small meals instead of three large ones. Remember to drink plenty of fluid. If you wait until you are thirsty, you are probably already dehydrated. Stop periodically to drink some water and, of course, use the bathroom. You will need to maintain a healthy amount of amniotic fluid in the placenta. So keep drinking.

It goes without saying that smoking, drinking and drugs are out of the question. Your doctor can help you quit if you have trouble on your own. A healthy baby is worth all the effort and sacrifice.

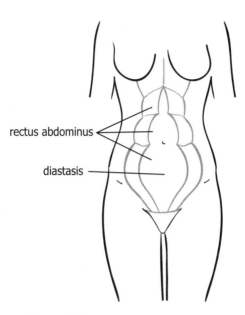

rectus abdominus

diastasis

FIGURE 6. **Diastasys**

How to use this book

Use this book as a pregnancy and fitness workbook. Throughout the book and at the end of each workout, you will find journal pages and diary-type questions for you to keep track of your pregnancy. There is also a space on each page for your own exercise notes. Did you do this exercise today? How many times did you perform this exercise this week? How did your body feel today? Was it easier/harder today? Why? How did your baby respond?

Each exercise has a **GOAL** and **PRENATAL BENEFIT** highlighted so that you can easily discover why you are doing each exercise and what you can hope to get out of it.

At the top of each exercise, there is a fun fact or reminder about your pregnancy or postpartum period. Some of them deal with nutrition while others point out milestones for your growing fetus or baby.

Also at the top of each exercise are the numbers ⚠1 ⚠2 ⚠3 ⚠4 ⚠5. One or more will be highlighted; these indicate the fitness level of the person who should do each exercise—a 1 being a beginner and a 5 being the advanced fitness or **Pilates** student. Remember to take other factors into account when assessing your fitness level. Is this your first pregnancy? You don't know yet how your body handles being pregnant. Are you over 35? There are increased risk factors for premature labor. Have you sustained any injuries in the past five years? Your body may still have weaknesses that need to be addressed.

All of these factors will lower your fitness level. Keep in mind that this isn't the time to get in the best shape of your life. It's the time to focus on giving your body the tools for a healthy and comfortable pregnancy and delivery. Your level may change from day to day. Make a note in the book when you have had to modify an exercise or skip it all together on that particular day and why. If you have done **Pilates** for years but are feeling very fatigued,

lower your level from a 5 to a 3. If you are combating morning sickness, start at a 1 or a 2. You can always increase the intensity later. Reevaluate your body everyday, accepting that your body will keep changing. Unlike a pre-pregnancy workout where the level of difficulty will keep increasing, the prenatal workout tends to lower the level of difficulty as your pregnancy progresses.

Pay attention to the comments set off by this exclamation mark symbol. There are certain movements that done incorrectly could put your body at risk for strain. If you find that you are doing what you have been warned to avoid, stop the exercise. Above all, listen to your body.

Note that many exercises have modifications allowing a broader range of people to participate. If you are unsure, are a beginner or are having trouble doing the regular exercise, please follow the modified version. Remember that as your baby grows, each exercise will become more difficult. Which means you will probably continue with the modified version even though you are actually getting stronger.

Whether you are pregnant or working out with your baby, you may need to pause or even stop from time to time. Even though **fluidity** (see Terms and Techniques) is an important element of the **Pilates Method**, your ability to sustain an unbroken flow of movement during pregnancy and postpartum will change our approach to this concept. You will need to get a drink and use the bathroom at least once during your workout, and you'll likely need to feed and calm a fussy baby (during the Post-natal workout). It's all right. Try to make the time you *are* exercising a smooth, choreographed dance.

The transition, or how you move from one exercise to the next, is as important as the actual exercise. Even though the exercises have been designed to be a continuous unbroken chain of movements, you may need only to do the exercises that work for a level 1, which means you may have to skip forward several pages in this book. If you are working at level 1 (or selecting among individual exercises), still transition out of the exercise you were just doing as if going into the next exercise in the book. Then, go to the transition on the page just prior to the exercise you are jumping to and pick up there so that you transition smoothly into the exercise you have chosen.

Attention to **flow** is very important while you are pregnant. It will keep you from jarring your body and moving suddenly or without thought. When you *do* pause or stop, please do it slowly and maintain your mind-body connection. If you are lying down, roll onto your left side and slowly sit up. Always transition back into the routine with an inhalation to get you into position. This flow will help your routine to leave you feeling relaxed, just as it does for the majority of **Pilates'** followers.

I have tried to word this book much in the same way I would speak to you in a one-on-one session. I have placed **helpful hints** next to the **execution** to add extra insight into the proper execution of the exercises so that you can reap the greatest rewards.

Ideally, you have the companion videos to this book. The **Prenatal Pilates** video and the **Post-natal Pilates** video are available through stores and at **www.pilatesforyou.com**. These products may help enlighten you even further into the way an exercise should be executed. There is a lot to absorb. Each time you read the book, watch the video and perform the exercise you may hear something you had missed before.

If you are lucky enough to find a certified **Pilates** *instructor who will work with you one-on-one, all the better. However,* **Prenatal Pilates** *is very new, so finding a certified teacher trained in* **Prenatal Pilates** *work may be difficult. Take the book with you. Nothing in this book is far from the norm, but the variations and trimester modifications are unique.*

Terms And Techniques

Although the human body is made up of thousands of muscles, tendons, ligaments, bones and arteries, I have highlighted only the larger ones that pertain most directly to **Pilates** and pregnancy and the ones you will hear most often talked about by instructors.

Under *Techniques*, I have described in greater detail a few very basic and important techniques that you will want to master before even beginning the actual exercises.

MUSCLES IN THE FRONT AND BACK OF THE BODY (FIGURES 7 & 8)

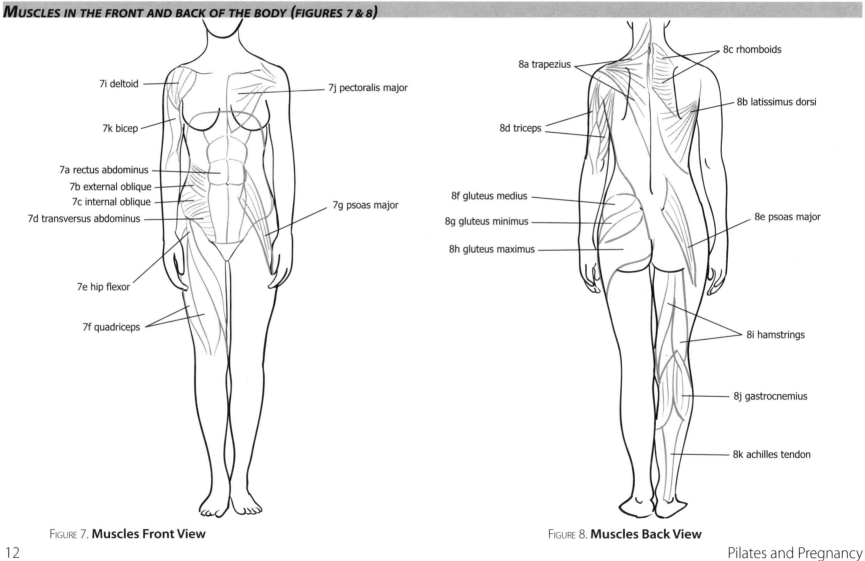

7i deltoid
7j pectoralis major
7k bicep
7a rectus abdominus
7b external oblique
7c internal oblique
7d transversus abdominus
7g psoas major
7e hip flexor
7f quadriceps

8a trapezius
8c rhomboids
8b latissimus dorsi
8d triceps
8f gluteus medius
8g gluteus minimus
8h gluteus maximus
8e psoas major
8i hamstrings
8j gastrocnemius
8k achilles tendon

FIGURE 7. **Muscles Front View**

FIGURE 8. **Muscles Back View**

ABDOMEN: There are four groups of muscles that comprise the abdominal wall. They are layered on top of each other.

1. **Rectus Abdominus** *(Figure 7a)*: The top most muscle layer that runs down the center of the body from ribs to pelvis. This is the muscle we think of giving us a "six pack." It is also the muscle most people utilize in abdominal work. This muscle is really two halves, joined by a seam. They can separate (**diastasys**) (Figure 6) during late pregnancy when they are over stretched or over worked. When the muscle doesn't heal properly, the contents of the abdomen can push through, leaving the woman with the tell tale pooch.

2. **External Oblique** *(Figure 7b)*: These muscles comprise the second layer and run diagonally from the ribcage on one side of your body to the opposite hip. When you cough or laugh, you can feel these muscles activate. They are very important for aiding in respiration (breathing) and keeping the **ribcage** from hyperextending (sticking out).

3. **Internal Oblique** *(Figure 7c)*: These lie under the **External Obliques** and run from the hips diagonally up to the ribcage. Both sets of **Obliques** work as a complimentary team; they are the muscles associated with a cinched waistline.

4. **Transversus Abdominus** *(Figure 7d)*: This is the deepest, most underused and certainly most important muscle. It runs in a sideways path from one hip to the other, and from the pubic bone to the belly button. This is the muscle that will provide core strength for your **powerhouse** as well as protection for your back. Finding this muscle is very difficult. Concentrate on pulling the muscles in from the inside rather than bearing down from the outside. I think of it like a **Kegal** that draws energy in and up the body. If you think of

---

*At no time are your abdominals to push out. You want to feel as though your transversus wraps around to your back connecting at your spine. At the same time, your back muscles wrap around to your belly button and lace up on the inside of your body. You'll often hear the phrase "**naval to spine**" (Figure 9) in Pilates. This is a way to train your muscles to lie flat while protecting your back. If you don't master this abdominal control, you may as well be doing traditional sit ups. Even as your uterus grows, you want the muscles to hug and support the baby during the exercises.

---

contracting the muscle you will inadvertently push the abdominal wall out, away from your back. The feeling you're looking for is more like a continuous motion to pull the belly toward the spine.

However, it is also important that you learn to release your muscles. Delivery requires energizing one muscle while relaxing another. While the **transversus** and the **obliques** are activated during pushing, the **pelvic floor** must release. You must rest all your muscles between contractions to conserve energy. You will also find your body reacting to the contractions with neck, shoulder and face tension. The more you can release this kind

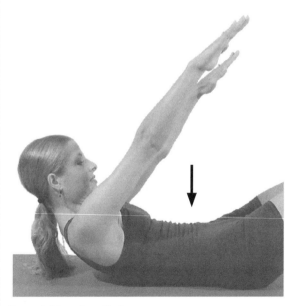

Figure 9. **Navel to Spine**

of muscle tension during contractions, the more comfortable you will be. Tension contributes to pain. No one wants that!

Bicep Muscle: *(Figure 7k)* The muscle in the front of the upper arm used to bend it.

Diaphragm *(Figure 10):* This large half balloon-like muscle aids in respiration by dropping down into the abdomen and making room for the lungs to expand.

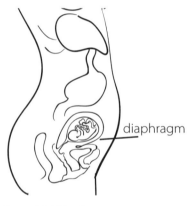

Figure 10. **Diaphragm**

Hamstring Muscle *(Figure 8i):* The large muscle in the back of the thigh is used to bend the leg.

Hip Flexors *(Figure 7e):* These muscles connect the torso to the legs. They are used to raise the leg and bend the torso forward.

Pelvic Floor *(Figure 11):* These are the muscles of the urethra, vagina and anus. They aid in supporting the bladder and uterus. They are the muscles used in **Kegel** exercises.

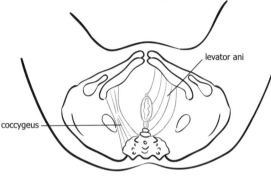

Figure 11. **Pelvic Floor**

Powerhouse *(Figure 1)* : This is a term refers to the muscles in your mid to low abdominal muscles and back. Almost every exercise is initiated here, and consequently almost all the exercises work to flatten and strengthen the stomach and fortify the back.

Quadricep Muscle *(Figure 7f):* This large muscle in the front of the thigh is used to straighten the leg.

Tricep Muscle *(Figure 8d):* The muscle in the back of your arm is used to straighten your arm

Coccyx/Tailbone *(Figure 13a):* The term refers to last bone/**vertebrae** in your spine.

Hip Bones *(Figure 12b):* The term identifies two bones on the front of your hips. They are actually the top of your **pelvis**.

Pelvis *(Figure 12c):* This is the group of bones that protects your uterus and bladder. It makes trianglular shape from your hips to your **pubic bone**.

Pubic Bone *(Figure 12a):* This is the bone at the base of your pelvis. Run your hand down the center of your stomach, the first bone you hit is your pubic bone. It may feel a little tender toward the end of your pregnancy.

Ribcage *(Figure 12d & 13d):* These are the bones that wrap around your torso and connect to your spine. They protect your lungs and heart. They are able to move sideways with each breath. They are also able to increase the space between one another to make room for your internal organs latter in pregnancy.

Shoulder Blades/Scapula *(Figure 13e):* These are the two bones of your upper back, referred to as "chicken wings".

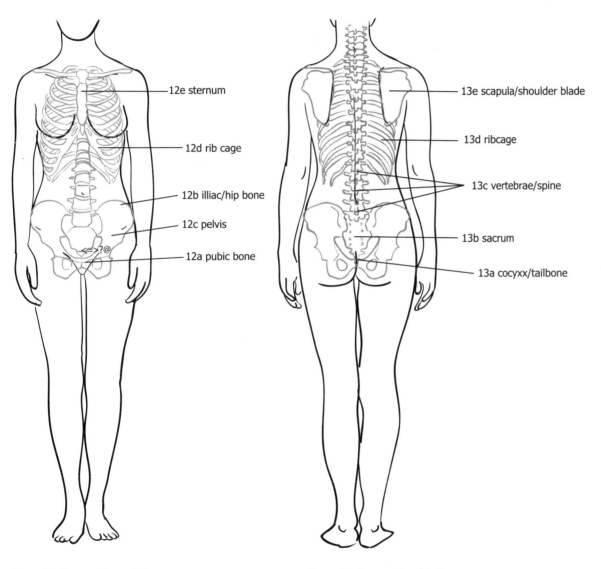

12e sternum

12d rib cage

12b illiac/hip bone

12c pelvis

12a pubic bone

13e scapula/shoulder blade

13d ribcage

13c vertebrae/spine

13b sacrum

13a cocyxx/tailbone

FIGURE 12. **Bones Front View**

FIGURE 13. **Bones Back View**

Spine (Figure 13c): There are twenty-six vertebrae in your back and neck.

Sternum (Figure 12e): Run your fingers up your ribcage. The place where they meet is your sternum.

Vertebrae (Figure 13c): These are the round bones on your spine. There are twenty-six in all starting at the base of your skull and ending with your tailbone. The more they can work independently, the healthier your back will be. When the **vertebrae** fuse together, you end up with back pain. Almost everyone has a stuck spot that will have to be slowly worked open. Therefore, only do part of an exercise; don't try to force yourself past a stuck section of spine. If, for instance, you cannot get each **vertebra** on the floor and keep the belly drawn in as you roll up to sitting, then only come part way up. To struggle through these tight places will only lead to back pain. Give it time, your back will become more flexible with dedication to proper form.

TECHNIQUES

Articulating the spine *(Figure 14):* Moving each **vertebra** one at a time in sequential order from the top to the bottom or the bottom to the top.

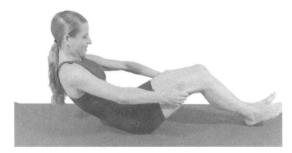

FIGURE 14. **Articulating**

Breathing *(Figure 15):* This will be the hardest yet most important concept to grasp. When we breathe naturally, our stomach rises and falls to make room for the **diaphragm. Pilates**

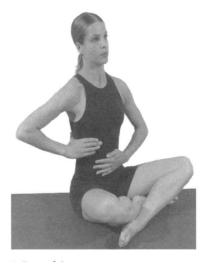

FIGURE 15. **Breathing**

breathing asks you to keep your stomach flat, while inhaling. Think of breathing into your lower back. This forces the ribcage to move sideways and backwards to accommodate the lungs and **diaphragm**. The intercostals or tendons that connect the ribs to one and other will slowly stretch allowing your lungs to fill to greater and greater capacity. This **breathing technique** helps ensure that your abdominals are always active and working to protect your back. In **Pilates,** you will always inhale through your nose and exhale out your mouth. You must exhale completely, "wringing out the lungs" so that no stale air is left and there is more room for a new breath. With few exceptions, you exhale on a muscle contraction, like bending forward from the hips, and inhale to prepare for an exercise and when the muscle lengthens or extends.

Chair Position *(Figure 16):* Lying on your back with your feet off the floor. Your legs make a ninety-degree angle.

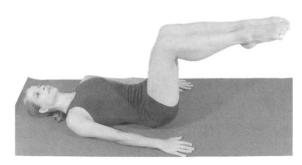

FIGURE 16. **Chair Position**

Contrology: The name **Joseph Pilates** gave his **Method**.

Fluidity: This is one of the major components of Joseph Pilates' method of "**Contrology**". At no time do you want to make jerky motions. **Pilates** is based on the flow from one movement to another. If you cannot do an exercise without a preparatory "heave," then only do part of it until you are stronger or more flexible. Sharp jerky motions and quick position changes can cause you to feel sharp ligament pain on one side of your belly. Stopping abruptly or getting up too quickly can also leave you feeling dizzy or lightheaded. MOVE SLOWLY!

Imprinting *(Figure 17):* This **Pilates** technique is how you allow your spine to be long and on the floor. Imagine that you are at the beach. You feel so relaxed that your spine melts into the sand. You don't push your spine down. Simply grow long in the torso and allow your spine room to reach for the floor. If your legs are bent, gravity will make this process easier. Imprinting will help keep your back from arching unsafely during the exercises.

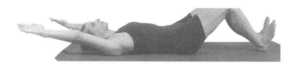

FIGURE 17. **Imprinting**

Pilates and Pregnancy

Kegel: This is a series of contraction and release exercises for the **pelvic floor.** Practice squeezing only the muscles of your vagina and anus. To find these muscles, practice stopping your flow of urine and at the same time, imagining that you are preventing gas from escaping. Your thighs and abdomen are not involved. Contract and release ten times up to four times a day. Try to work up to fifty repetitions four times a day. It is important to release. The strength built from contracting will help with incontinence while the ability to fully release will aid in child birth.

Legs hip-width apart *(Figures 18a, 18b, 18c, 18d):* While lying on your back, find your correct alignment by starting with your legs and feet together (a). Turn your toes in and heels out (b). Bring your toes in line with your heels (c). Then open your knees in line with your feet (d).

Navel to spine *(Figure 9):* This is a Pilates technique, in which you concentrate on drawing your abdomen toward your back in order to keep your powerhouse active and imprint your spine on the floor.

Neutral Pelvis *(Figure 19):* This term means that your pelvis is neither tucked nor arched and your tailbone is on the floor. Unless otherwise indicated, your pelvis will always start and finish in this position when you are lying on your back. There may be a slight space under your lower back when your legs are straight.

However, you are always **imprinting.** Remaining in **neutral pelvis** trains the abdominal muscles to grow strong in the position you will be in while standing. Almost everyone has a natural curve in the lower back; however, this can be exaggerated in pregnancy

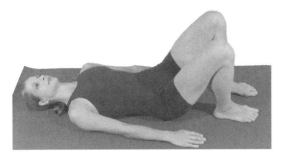

FIGURE 19. **Neutral pelvis**

due to the weight of the uterus. Therefore it is important to stay in a true neutral. To find this, place the heel of your hands on your **hip bones** and your middle fingers on your **pubic bone.** They should be even. If the pubic bone is above the hips you are tucked, if it is below the hips you are arched. It is just as important to recognize the tucked position since you will have to go through this position any time you roll through the spine.

Pelvic Tilt *(Figure 20):* You will always go through a least a small **pelvic tilt** while articulating your spine. However you want to release it at the start or finish of the exercise.

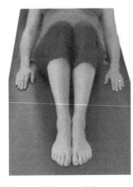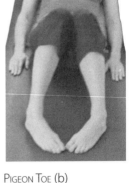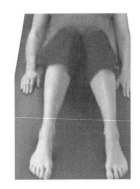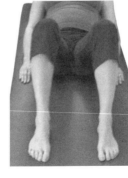

STARTING POSITION (a)   PIGEON TOE (b)   TOES IN LINE WITH HEALS (c)   KNEES IN LINE WITH FEET (d)

FIGURE 18. **Bringing legs hip-width apart**

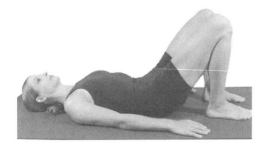

FIGURE 20. **Pelvic Tilt**

Edema: Swelling

Diastasys (Figure 6): A separation of the rectus abdominus muscle. This often occurs during pregnancy as the muscle becomes overstretched.

Varicosities/varicose veins: Swelling and enlargement of the veins, commonly seen in the legs. These can develop as a result of weight gain, poor circulation and heredity.

Vena Cava (Figure 4): A major artery that supplies blood to both you and your baby.

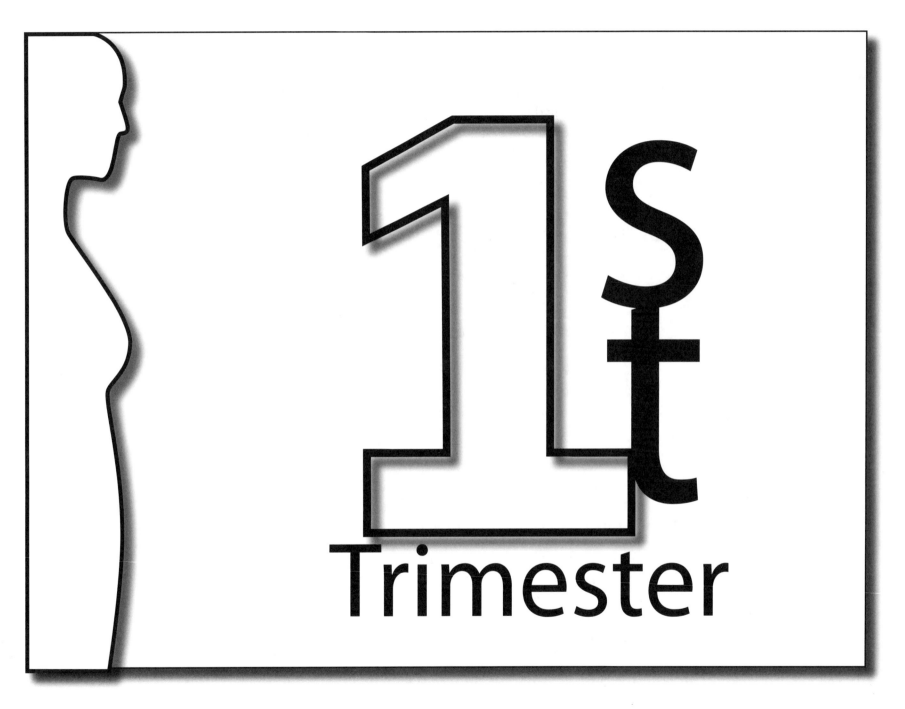

1st Trimester

First Trimester Workout

This first trimester workout is a great program to use if you are thinking about becoming pregnant and want to prepare your body. If you are starting this program after you have found out you are pregnant and have had your first visit with your doctor, there is really very little time left in the first trimester. Ideally you can continue these exercises until the end of your fourth month, but that depends on your comfort level while lying on your back.

This is the time to target and tone your abdominal wall. Make the most of it by really concentrating on what you are doing. You are going to feel tired and possibly nauseous, so take frequent breaks and drink plenty of water. Although it would be nice to get a workout in from beginning to end, that is not always possible or advisable. (See **How to Use This Book**).

To combat the nausea, have a light snack about a half hour before working out. Always keep crackers close by; they will be your friends when you're not feeling great. Make sure you have loose, comfortable clothes on. You don't need anything extra tight around your stomach. It will cause you to feel queasy.

Have water at hand and take frequent breaks to drink it. Be prepared to go to the bathroom often. Pregnancy hormones, lots of water and the deep abdominal work will all cause you to need to urinate frequently.

Above all, stop if you feel light headed or nauseous. You can always resume later. Don't try to work through it. You won't be able to concentrate fully, which will defeat the purpose. Keep a small towel close by and place two soup cans or three-pound weights next to a wall that you can lean against.

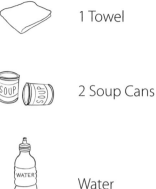

You will need:

1 Towel

2 Soup Cans

Water

1 Pillow

The pictures in this chapter are primarily of Kristine who is preparing her body for her first pregnancy.

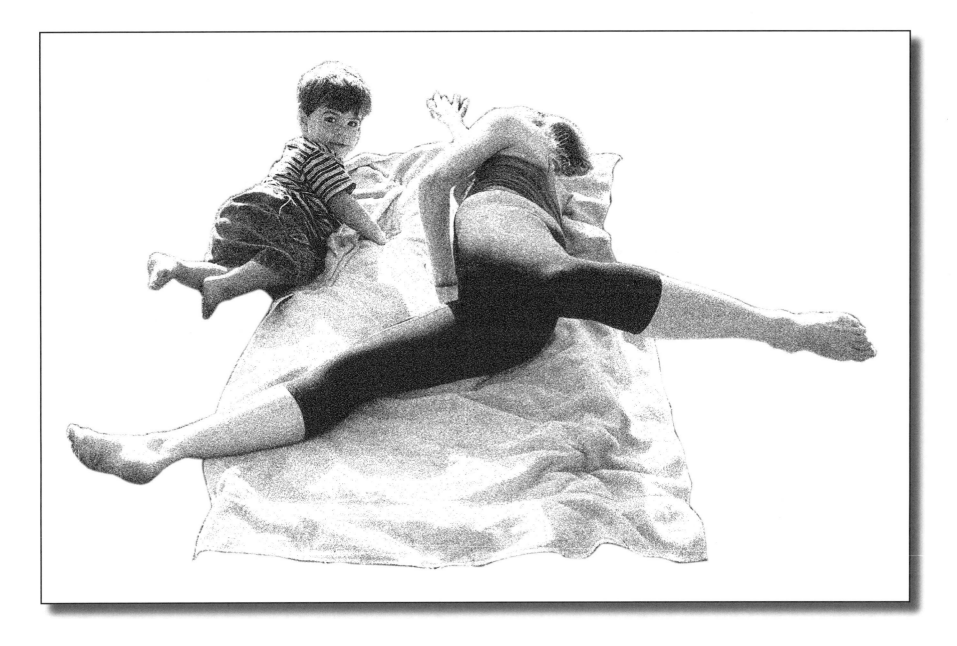

Breathing

What is needed:

WATER

NOTES:

GOAL: To learn to breath into your **ribcage** and lower back while not allowing your belly to rise and fall. This will increase the space between your ribs to allow for maximum air intake. The more you practice the **PILATES BREATHING,** the greater your lung capacity will be.

PRENATAL BENEFITS: Increased lung capacity equals increased endurance. Efficient breathing and endurance will help limit fatigue during labor. Deep breathing also helps in pain management. Think about what you do naturally when you are hurt. Stub your toe and you would likely take a deep sipping breath.

POSITION:

LIE on your back, knees bent, feet flat on the floor. Place one hand on your stomach, the other on the side of your **ribcage**. **Pelvis** is in neutral—neither tucked nor arched. Imprint your spine into the mat.

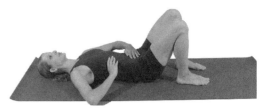

* *In Pilates you will always inhale through your nose and exhale out your mouth.*

EXECUTION:

BEGIN by breathing incorrectly a few times.

INHALE through your nose and let your stomach rise and pull away from your back. Exhale and let your stomach fall.

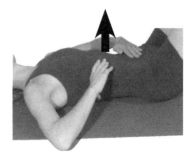

Incorrect

Helpful Hints:

As you inhale, feel your ribs move into your hand. Try to breath into your lower back. Imagine squeezing the air out of your lungs with your ribs as you exhale.

Be careful not to breathe into your shoulders. Keep your neck and shoulders relaxed and open.

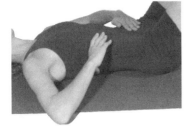

Now practice correct **PILATES BREATHING**.

INHALE through your nose, expanding your **ribcage** sideways and into the floor. Your stomach stays flat. Your back is **imprinted** on the floor.

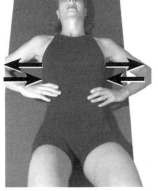

EXHALE out your mouth, squeezing your ribs together and drawing them down toward your hips.

Practice correct **PILATES BREATHING** *at least ten times.*

Try to remember this technique in all of your exercises.

Incorrect

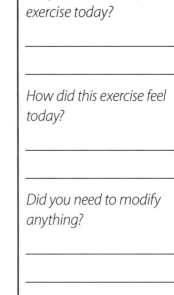

For your review:

Did you need to skip this exercise today?

_____

_____

How did this exercise feel today?

_____

_____

Did you need to modify anything?

_____

_____

Did your baby react more or less today?

_____

_____

TRANSITION:

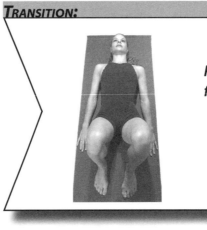

Place your arms on the floor at your sides.

Knee Folds

What is needed:

NOTES:

_____

_____

_____

_____

_____

Helpful Hints:

This is an abdominal exercise, not a leg workout, so initiate the movement from your **powerhouse**.

GOAL: To tone your **powerhouse** and train them to stay active so they can protect your spine.

PRENATAL BENEFITS: This kind of abdominal awareness before moving will become second nature in your day-to-day activities. Protecting your back from further arching will be crucial in limiting lower back strains.

POSITION:

LIE on your back, feet flat on the floor **hip-width apart**. To ensure proper foot/leg placement, refer to Terms and Techniques. Your shoulders are wide and down. Your hands are at your sides and slightly pressing into the floor.

EXECUTION:

INHALE to prepare. While keeping your hips still, exhale and float your right leg to a ninety-degree angle.

INHALE at the top.

EXHALE as you float your left leg up to **chair position**. It is crucial to keep your stomach flat and reaching for your spine while maintaining a **neutral pelvis**.

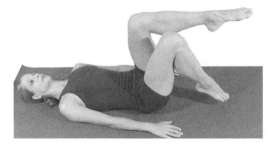

INHALE as you lower your right leg. Draw your abdominal muscles in and up so that your **powerhouse** remains tight and active.

EXHALE at the bottom.

INHALE to lower your left leg.

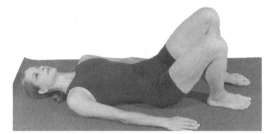

EXHALE as your foot touches the floor.

This completes one set.

Do three sets, alternating legs.

Do one more but keep your legs in chair position.

TRANSITION:

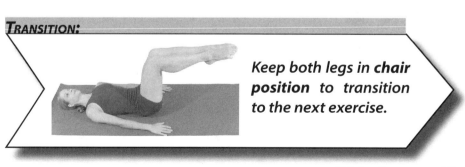

Keep both legs in chair position to transition to the next exercise.

THE moment your stomach sticks out or the arch in your lower back increases, stop and try again.

The Hundred

What is needed:

NOTES:

_____

_____

_____

_____

_____

*This is the signature exercise of **Pilates**. If you only have time for one exercise, do this one. It works on so many things at once. It gets your circulation going, tones your abdominal muscles and builds stamina.*

GOAL: To increase blood circulation and strengthen your **powerhouse**.

PRENATAL BENEFITS: Blood volume almost doubles in pregnancy. It is important to stimulate your circulation so that blood doesn't pool in your legs, which can cause **edema** and **varicose** or spider veins.

POSITION:

LIE on your back with both legs together and bent at a ninety-degree angle in **chair position**. **Pelvis** is in **neutral**. Your arms reach long, drawing your shoulders down your back, as if your fingers were trying to touch the wall in front of you.

INHALE as your head and shoulders curl off the floor. Leave space for a small orange to fit under your chin. Your lower back should remain in contact with the floor as you exhale and extend your legs toward the ceiling or slightly past ninety-degrees. Your legs are turned out from your hip and your heels are together. Reach your arms long and allow them to float about two inches off the floor.

Helpful Hints:

Remember to expand your ribs sideways and back so that your stomach stays still as it did for BREATHING.

Only your arms move in this exercise; your torso and legs remain stable.

Keep your legs long.

The movement is initiated from your **shoulder blades** not your lower arms or hands.

Your arms are a metronome for your breath.

If your stomach pushes out or the arch in your lower back increases, return to **chair position**.

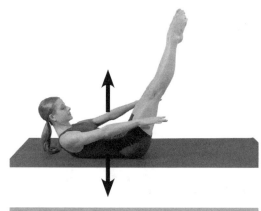

EXECUTION:

PUMP your arms up and down with resistance as if you were under water.

INHALE slowly for five counts. Then exhale slowly for five counts.

This is one set.

Do ten sets.

MODIFICATION:

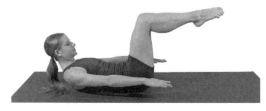

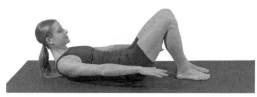

You can begin with five sets and work your way up to ten if you don't have the stamina yet to do all ten.

This exercise can be done with your legs together and bent in **chair position** or with your feet together and flat on the floor. Go to where you can control your abdominals and keep your back from arching.

TRANSITION:

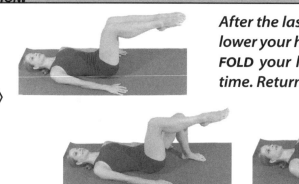

*After the last set, bend your legs and lower your head and shoulders. KNEE FOLD your legs back down one at a time. Return to a **hip-width** position.*

For your review:

Did you need to skip this exercise today?

_____

_____

How did this exercise feel today?

_____

_____

Did you need to modify anything?

_____

_____

Did your baby react more or less today?

_____

_____

Bridging

What is needed:

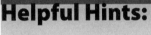

GOAL: To increase your spine's mobility by moving each **vertebra** separately.

PRENATAL BENEFITS: **BRIDGING** helps stretch the front of your thighs and hips as well as your back. It relieves the exaggerated arch in the lower back that tends to occur during pregnancy. This is one exercise that feels so good you'll want to do it often!

NOTES:

_____

_____

_____

_____

POSITION:

LIE on your back, knees bent, feet flat on the floor, **hip-width** apart. Arms at your sides, shoulders relaxed and wide on the floor. Reach your fingers toward your feet to keep your neck long.

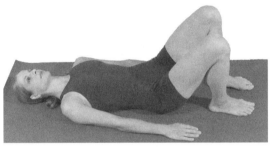

Helpful Hints:

Reach your arms down to keep your neck long.

Your inner thighs should pull toward each other to counteract the desire to roll out on your feet.

Thinking of the front of your body will help you keep from arching.

EXECUTION:

INHALE and tilt your **pelvis** up by pulling your abdominal muscles into your spine and your lower back into the floor. Your **pubic bone** will curl up toward your belly button.

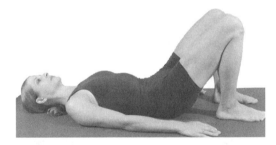

EXHALE as you continue to peel one **vertebra** off the floor at a time by pulling your abdominal muscles into your spine and tilting your **pelvis** up until you reach your shoulders. You should be in one line from your knees to your shoulders.

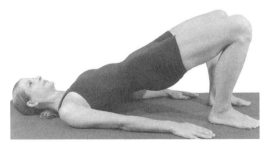

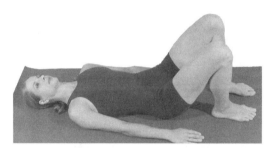

Inhale to soften your **sternum** into the floor while keeping your **buttocks** lifted.

Exhale as you continue to melt the front of your body into the floor until you are all the way back to **neutral**.

This is one set.

Do four sets.

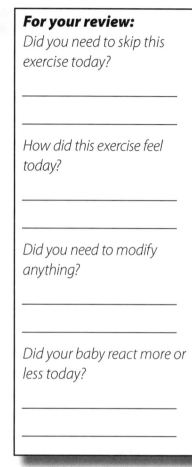

For your review:

Did you need to skip this exercise today?

_____

_____

How did this exercise feel today?

_____

_____

Did you need to modify anything?

_____

_____

Did your baby react more or less today?

_____

_____

Transition:

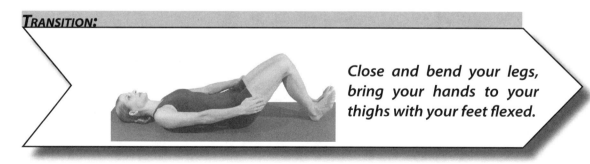

Close and bend your legs, bring your hands to your thighs with your feet flexed.

Stop–n–Go

△3 △4 △5

What is needed:

NOTES:

_____

_____

_____

_____

Helpful Hints:

This is a great warm-up for ROLL UP.

It is very important that you keep your **navel to spine** in so that your back can round.

Really hold onto your legs so your can pull your back into a "C" curve.

GOAL: To locate and tone weak sections in your abdominal wall while isolating and opening stuck sections of your spine.

PRENATAL BENEFITS: This exercise is a variation of ROLL UP and helps counteract lower back discomfort that can develop during pregnancy. This exercise targets each section of abdominal muscle and helps train your **obliques** to support your growing uterus and the **transversus** to support your internal organs (especially your bladder). This is the time to train and tone your **rectus** so that it will return to a tighter and flatter position after pregnancy.

POSITION:

LIE on your back with your legs bent and your hands behind your thighs. Use your hands to help pull you up. This is an easier way to do a ROLL UP, yet it is more intense since you can use your legs as a counter balance to really draw the belly in.

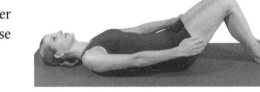

EXECUTION:

EXHALE to round your head and shoulders off the floor.

INHALE to stay and pull your abdominal wall in.

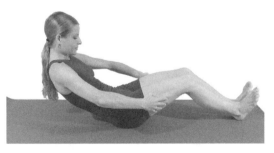

EXHALE and round up a little higher to about mid back.

INHALE as you stay and pull your abdominal muscles in and up even more. Feel your **obliques** wrap around you and melt through your belly button into your spine.

Pilates and Pregnancy

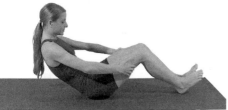

EXHALE as you come up a little higher so that only your lower back touches the floor.

INHALE to stay and pull your abdominal muscles in and up even more. Make sure your **pelvi**s is fully tilted up so that your lower back is on the floor.

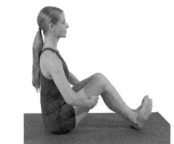

EXHALE to curl the rest of the way up. Stay rounded in your spine and straighten your legs with feet flexed and reach toward your toes. Keep your shoulders down and your back rounded. Your belly should be pulled in.

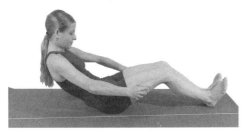

INHALE to sit tall and soften your knees. Place your hands behind your thighs.

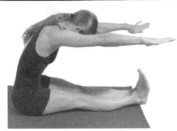

EXHALE and tuck your **pelvis** under. Pull your belly away from your thighs and roll all the way down to the floor.

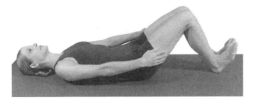

INHALE to finish in the starting position.

This is one set.

Do six sets.

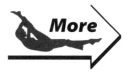 **More**

MODIFICATION:

As with **ROLL UP**, if you cannot keep your **navel to spine** and get each part of your back on the floor, only do the first two increments, coming only to your mid back.

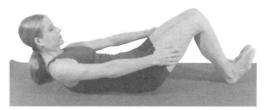

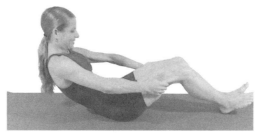

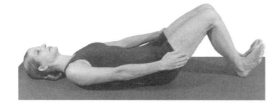

TRANSITION:

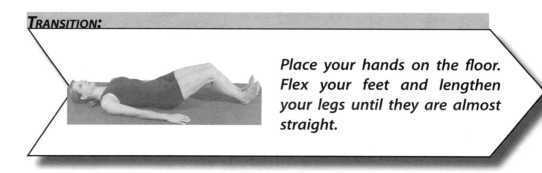

Place your hands on the floor. Flex your feet and lengthen your legs until they are almost straight.

FINDING OUT I'M PREGNANT

The day I found out I… _____

_____

_____

_____

_____

_____

My first visit to the doctor… _____

_____

_____

_____

_____

When I saw you for the first time in the sonogram… _____

_____

_____

_____

_____

Roll Up

What is needed:

[water bottle illustration] WATER

NOTES:

_____

_____

_____

_____

GOAL: To stretch your back and legs while using your **powerhouse**.

PRENATAL BENEFITS: Finding the deep abdominal muscles that will be used during delivery is crucial for developing the muscle memory that will be needed when you are so over stretched you won't feel like you have muscles.

Traditionally this exercise is done with completely straight legs, but it is very hard for anyone to do this exercise correctly and still make sure the lower back does not get strained. Pregnant women have an even harder time getting their lower back to round, so I encourage all women to have their knees at least slightly bent. The degree of bend in your legs depends on your abdominal strength and back flexibility.

POSITION:

LIE on your back with your feet flexed and legs together long and slightly bent.

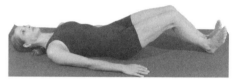

INHALE as you take your arms toward the ceiling, exhale and bring them over your head. Keep your ribs down. Do not touch the floor with your hands when they are over your head or your back will pull away from the floor.

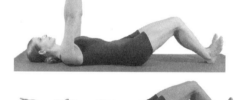

Helpful Hints:

As your arms reach over head, your ribs reach toward your hips.

Pull your inner thighs together.

As you roll up, if you feel yourself get stuck and unable to round more, stop and hold your legs so that you can pull your belly in even more. This will help you tease your back open.

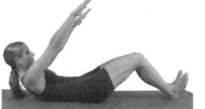

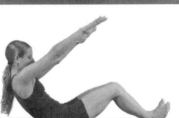

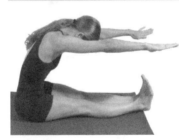

EXECUTION:

INHALE to curl your head and shoulders off the floor while keeping your head between your arms.

EXHALE and continue rolling up, one **vertebra** at a time. Make sure your abdominal muscles reach toward your spine.

STRAIGHTEN your legs at the top and reach your body forward as if lying over a beach ball, again keeping your head between your arms.

INHALE as you start to roll down allowing your **pelvis** to tuck under and your lower back to reach into the floor.

EXHALE and continue to uncurl one **vertebra** at a time until you are back to the starting position. Keep your arms over your head.

This is one set.

Do six sets.

! If you feel stress in your lower back and cannot pull your lower back into the floor on the way up or down, stop and do the modification.

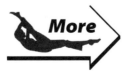

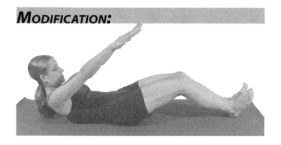

Modification: Only come part way up but really concentrate on keeping your belly drawn in and your head between your arms. As you become stronger and the space between your **vertebrae** increases, you will be able to come up higher.

For your review:

Did you need to skip this exercise today?

_____

_____

How did this exercise feel today?

_____

_____

Did you need to modify anything?

_____

_____

Did your baby react more or less today?

_____

_____

_____

TRANSITION:

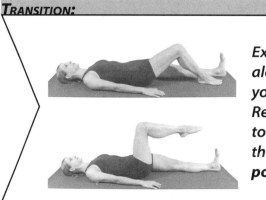

Extend your left leg along the floor with your foot still flexed. Relax your right foot to the floor. KNEE FOLD the right leg to chair position.

THOUGHTS AND FEELINGS

Date: _____

This time in my pregnancy has been… _____

_____

_____

_____

_____

_____

I feel good about my body because… _____

_____

_____

_____

_____

I am anxious about… _____

_____

_____

_____

_____

Leg Circles

What is needed:

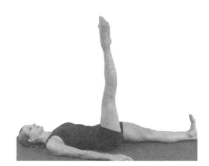

WATER

NOTES:

_____

_____

_____

Helpful Hints:

This is an abdominal exercise!

Relaxing your foot helps keep your thigh from engaging.

Really reach your standing leg away. It will help stabilize your torso.

Your torso and hips should not move.

GOAL: To learn to move your leg independently from the rest of your body.

PRENATAL BENEFITS: Having one leg in the air can help let fluid and blood drain from your legs where it tends to pool. Circling your leg increases circulation.

POSITION:

LIE on your back with your arms straight, palms pressing lightly into the floor at your sides. Your left leg is extended along the floor, foot flexed. Extend your right leg to the ceiling and turn your leg out from the hip. Your foot is relaxed. Your arms are at your sides with your palms pressing into the floor. Your **pelvis** is in **neutral.** Your shoulders are wide and down, and your neck is relaxed.

EXECUTION:

MAKE tiny circles in the air with your leg by crossing your leg over the center of your body, taking your leg down and around and up. Keep your navel reaching for your spine. Try to initiate the motion from your **powerhouse,** not your thigh. Eventually your leg will feel light.

INHALE for half the circle. Exhale for half and pause at the top.

Make five circles in one direction.

Reverse the circle and do five more in the opposite direction.

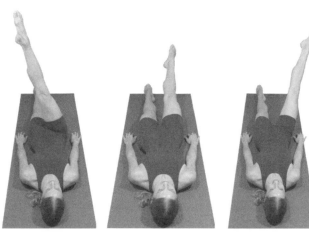

Cross the center of your body.

Bring your leg down slowly.

Open just past your hips and return to the starting position.

Pause at the top.

FOLIC ACID IS ESPECIALLY IMPORTANT BEFORE AND DURING THE FIRST 3 MONTHS OF PREGNANCY.

For your review:

Did you need to skip this exercise today?

_____

_____

How did this exercise feel today?

_____

_____

Did you need to modify anything?

_____

_____

Did your baby react more or less today?

_____

_____

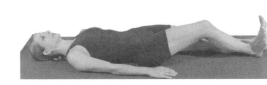

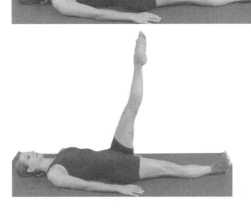

SWITCH sides:

BRING your right leg back to center, bend it and lower it to the ground. Flex your right foot and reach your leg long along the floor.

POINT your left foot and draw your left leg back in. KNEE FOLD your leg to **chair position** and extend your foot and leg, turned out, to the ceiling.

Do five circles in both directions on your left leg.

MODIFICATION:

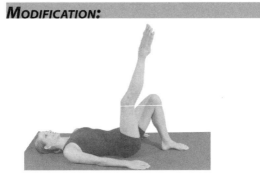

If your legs or back are tight bend one or both legs.

TRANSITION:

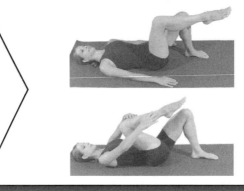

*Bend your left or working leg to **chair position** and place your foot flat on the floor. Bend your right leg and float it to **chair position**. Place your right hand on your right ankle and your left hand on your knee.*

Stomach Series

What is needed:

NOTES:

_____

_____

_____

_____

_____

The stomach series is designed to target all four abdominal muscle groups.
There are five exercises in the series. We will do the first two.

GOAL: To strengthen your powerhouse.

PRENATAL BENEFITS: The first trimester is the best time to work your abdominal muscles intensely. The deep strength developed will aid in delivery while the muscle memory built will help train your muscles to return to a flatter and stronger shape after pregnancy.

Single Leg Stretch   △3 △4 △5

POSITION:

LIE on your back with your right leg bent toward your chest and your left leg extended, reaching at a forty-five-degree angle. Your right hand is on your right ankle; your left hand is on your right knee. Your head and shoulders are off the floor. Try to soften your neck and shoulders. Your **pelvis** is in **neutral**.

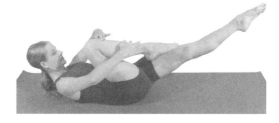

Helpful Hints:

Imagine that you are practicing kegels, so that you are working your abdominals from the inside.

If it is too hard to continue one breath through both legs, you can alternate your breath with your legs.

EXECUTION:

INHALE. Pull your right knee gently toward your chest with two pulses.

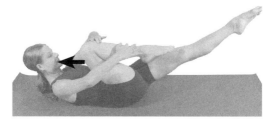

> ! YOUR lower back should not arch. It is best to err on the side of tucking to ensure your lower back remains on the floor and is protected.

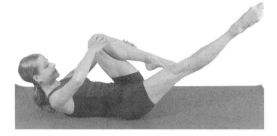

SWITCH legs and hands:

YOUR left hand goes on your left ankle, right hand goes on your left knee. Your right leg is extended. Your **powerhouse** stays drawn in and up.

This is one set.

Do eight sets.

Alternate your breath with each set. Inhale to do the first set; exhale to do the second, and so on until you complete all eight sets.

MODIFICATION:

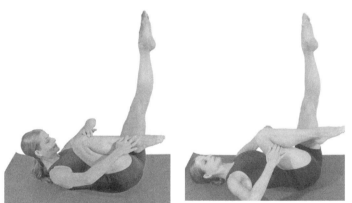

EXTEND your leg to the ceiling if your lower back pulls away from the floor.

IF your neck and shoulders feel strained, lower your head and shoulders. You can also take your hands behind your thighs.

! ONLY rest your head and shoulders on the floor if your extended leg also points to the ceiling.

TRANSITION:

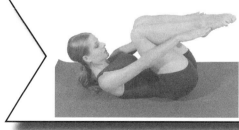

Bend both legs into your chest while reaching your hands to your ankles. Keep your head and shoulders rounded off the floor.

For your review:
Did you need to skip this exercise today?

_____

_____

How did this exercise feel today?

_____

_____

Did you need to modify anything?

_____

_____

Did your baby react more or less today?

_____

_____

What is needed:

NOTES:

_____

_____

_____

_____

Double Leg Stretch   △4 △5

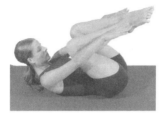

POSITION:

LIE on your back with both legs bent toward your chest, knees slightly apart and heels together and both hands reaching toward your ankles. Your head and shoulders stay curled off the floor throughout the exercise.

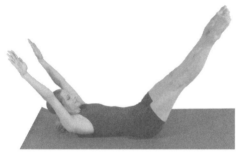

EXECUTION:

INHALE to extend your arms and legs on the diagonal in opposite directions without lowering your upper back. Your legs turn out as they extend. Keep your heels touching and reach your legs long. Again, your abdominal muscles are drawn in and up. Make sure your shoulders do not lift as your arms reach away.

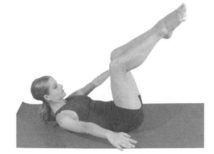

Helpful Hints:

Make sure your upper-back does not lower as your arms reach away.

Imprinting is essential to keep your back on the floor.

EXHALE as you bend your legs and circle your arms around to the starting position.

This is one set.

Do four sets.

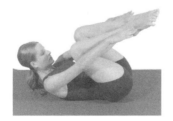

Pilates and Pregnancy

! Your stomach is going to want to push out. If your stomach pushes out, your back's safety will be compromised. You must use considerable effort to keep your back from arching more when you extend your legs. Do the modification if you feel your stomach push out or your back arch.

MODIFICATION:

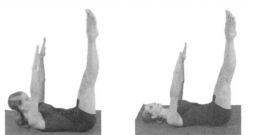

Extend your arms and legs directly to the ceiling if your back comes off the floor. In this position, it is also safe to lower your head and shoulders if you feel excessive strain in your neck. Your knees can be slightly bent.

For your review:

Did you need to skip this exercise today?

_____

_____

How did this exercise feel today?

_____

_____

Did you need to modify anything?

_____

_____

Did your baby react more or less today?

_____

_____

TRANSITION:

Lower your head and shoulders. Then lower your feet one at a time. Roll onto your left side with your left arm over your head, palm down on the floor, and your right palm on the floor directly in front of your sternum. Place a towel under your head for support and extend your legs. Flex your feet forward to a forty-five-degree angle while keeping your tailbone reaching back to avoid tucking.

Side Kick Series

What is needed:

NOTES:

_____

_____

_____

_____

_____

_____

This is a side lying leg series. There are many exercises in the series. We will only do two. First we will work one side and then the other.

GOAL: To stabilize your torso using your **powerhouse** so that you can move your leg freely, while stretching your **hip flexors**, lower back, **hamstrings and inner thighs.**

PRENATAL BENEFITS: Your growing belly and added weight will want to compress your body and shorten your muscles. This exercise will help train you to work with a longer torso and better posture even as your growing baby puts demands on your body.

Front/Back ⚠2 ⚠3 ⚠4 ⚠5

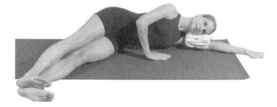

POSITION:

LIE on your left side with your legs parallel at a forty-five-degree angle from your body. Your feet are flexed. Your left arm is over your head with the palm down.

PLACE a rolled up towel under your head. Your right hand is on the floor in front of your **sternum**. It is very important to maintain the integrity of this position. Your back is straight and your **pelvis** in **neutral**. Feel as if you are sticking your buttocks

Helpful Hints:

Work in opposition. As your leg kicks front, your tailbone reaches down and a little back. As your leg kicks back, your abdominal muscles draw in and up and your ribs pull down.

Keeping your torso "still" doesn't mean it is inactive.

Note, this position will limit your range of motion. That's okay. Although your leg can go higher when your **pelvis** is tucked, that tucked **pelvis** compresses your body and actually takes some of the stretch away from your leg.

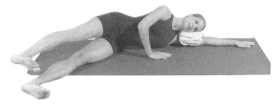

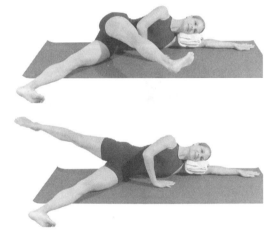

POSITION (CONTINUED):

out slightly to keep your **pelvis** from tucking. There will be a small, natural arch in your lower back.

KEEP your abdominal muscles and ribs pulled in to assist in maintaining this position. Your top shoulder and hip should be stacked directly on top of the underneath side.

WHILE keeping your bottom (left) leg straight and parallel with the foot flexed, inhale and release the top (right) leg to hip height. Moving your legs shouldn't affect your torso by rocking it forward or back nor by rounding or arching.

EXECUTION:

EXHALE as you kick to the front with a double pulse. Make sure the buttocks and back stay reaching long and down to allow your leg to truly stretch.

INHALE and point your foot as you reach your leg to the back.

This is one set.

Do eight sets

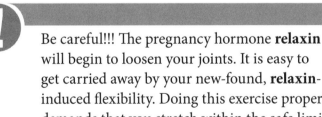

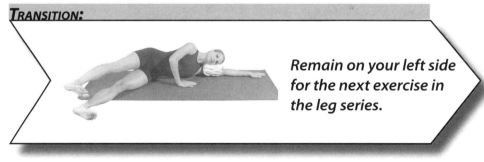

! Be careful!!! The pregnancy hormone **relaxin** will begin to loosen your joints. It is easy to get carried away by your new-found, **relaxin**-induced flexibility. Doing this exercise properly demands that you stretch within the safe limits of your body by not allowing you to wack your leg and pull a muscle. It teaches body control.

TRANSITION:

Remain on your left side for the next exercise in the leg series.

For your review:

Did you need to skip this exercise today?

_____

_____

How did this exercise feel today?

_____

_____

Did you need to modify anything?

_____

_____

Did your baby react more or less today?

_____

_____

Side Kick Series

What is needed:

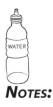

WATER

NOTES:

_____

_____

Helpful Hints:

Your top hip will want to roll back to give your leg a greater range of motion. Don't! If you give into this temptation, your flexibility will never improve.

Think of pressing your top hip slightly forward as you kick up to keep your hips stacked one on top of the other.

Your **pelvis** will want to tuck under. Reach your **tailbone** down to counteract it.

Keep your standing leg reaching long with your foot flexed.

Up/Down

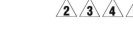

POSITION:

LYING on your left side, turn your right leg out place your right heel on the instep of your left foot. Point your right foot.

EXECUTION:

EXHALE and kick up to the side. Your torso stays long and doesn't rock back.

INHALE as you flex your foot and control your leg coming down.

This is one set.

Do eight sets.

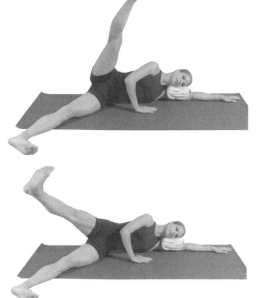

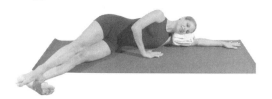

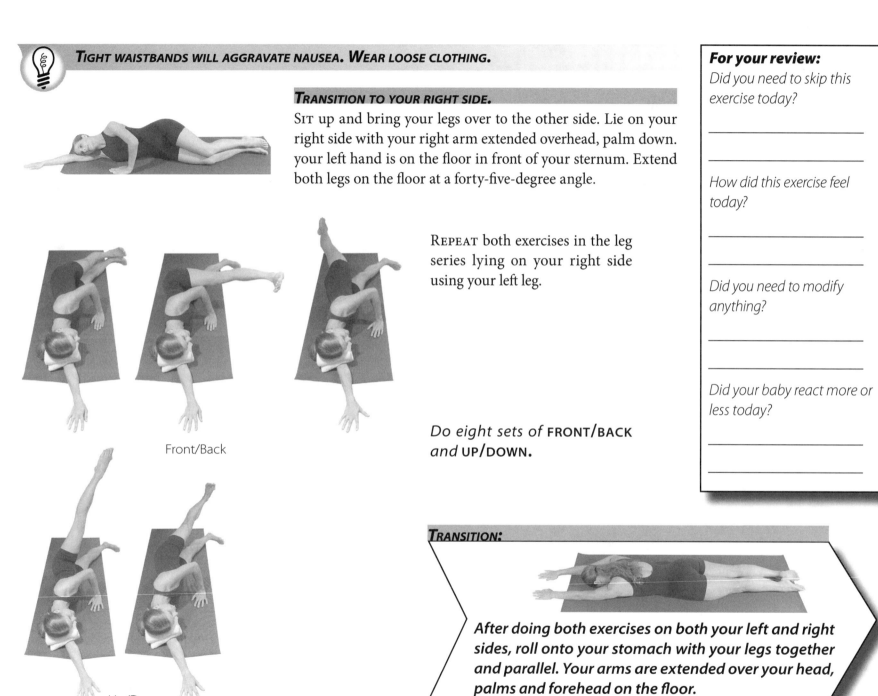

💡 **TIGHT WAISTBANDS WILL AGGRAVATE NAUSEA. WEAR LOOSE CLOTHING.**

TRANSITION TO YOUR RIGHT SIDE.

SIT up and bring your legs over to the other side. Lie on your right side with your right arm extended overhead, palm down. your left hand is on the floor in front of your sternum. Extend both legs on the floor at a forty-five-degree angle.

REPEAT both exercises in the leg series lying on your right side using your left leg.

Do eight sets of FRONT/BACK and UP/DOWN.

Front/Back

Up/Down

For your review:

Did you need to skip this exercise today?

_____

_____

How did this exercise feel today?

_____

_____

Did you need to modify anything?

_____

_____

Did your baby react more or less today?

_____

_____

TRANSITION:

After doing both exercises on both your left and right sides, roll onto your stomach with your legs together and parallel. Your arms are extended over your head, palms and forehead on the floor.

Swimming

What is needed:

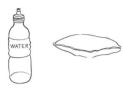

NOTES:

_____

_____

_____

GOAL: To strengthen the muscles in your back.

PRENATAL BENEFITS: During pregnancy, your upper back tends to round forward and your chest closes. This exercise helps open your chest and strengthen the muscles that draw your shoulders down your back, to improve your posture.

POSITION:

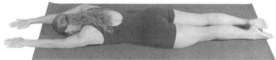

LIE on your stomach with your legs together and in parallel. Your arms are over your head with your palms and forehead on the floor. You are in a slight **pelvic tilt** to keep your lower back long and to take some pressure off your stomach. Lift your abdominal muscles into your back.

EXECUTION:

THERE ARE TWO PARTS TO THIS EXERCISE.
PART I IS A WARM UP.
PART II IS THE FULL SWIMMING EXERCISE.

Helpful Hints:

Your torso must remain imprinted as your arms and legs move.

Reaching your arm long first makes the muscle longer and lighter. Your shoulder must move in opposition to your arm to achieve this.

Imagine a string attached to your buttocks and back of your knee to keep your leg straight.

Find the strength between your **shoulder blades** so that your whole arm moves.

Recreational swimmers may have trouble with this exercise, since they are used to reaching with their shoulder when they stroke. Be patient! Learning to release your arm from your shoulder will give you more flexibility.

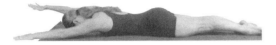

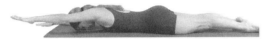

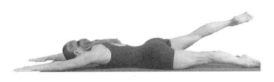

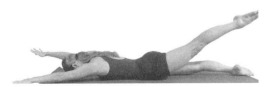

EXECUTION: PART I:

INHALE while reaching your right arm so far that it floats off the floor. Make sure your shoulder stays down and attached to your back.

EXHALE to lower your arm.

SWITCH arms:

INHALE to reach your left arm off the floor. Exhale to lower it down.

WITHOUT shifting your hips, inhale and reach your right leg so long that it floats off the ground.

EXHALE and lower your leg.

SWITCH legs.

INHALE to reach your left leg off the floor.

EXHALE to lower it down.

INHALE and lift your right arm and left leg, re aching them in opposite directions.

EXHALE and lower.

SWITCH sides and repeat with your left arm and right leg.

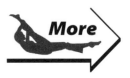

EXECUTION: PART II:

Now that you have warmed up and practiced lengthening your limbs without hip and shoulder distortions, do the full swimming exercise.

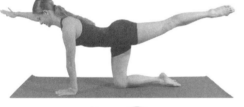

INHALE. Raise both arms, both legs and your head but keep your focus down to keep the back of your neck long.

ALTERNATE moving your arms and legs up and down as if swimming.

INHALE for two counts. Exhale for two counts.

This is one set.

Do four sets.

<table>
<tr><td>

For your review:

Did you need to skip this exercise today?

_____

_____

How did this exercise feel today?

_____

_____

Did you need to modify anything?

_____

_____

_____

Did your baby react more or less today?

_____

_____

</td></tr>
</table>

MODIFICATION:

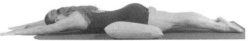

If you are uncomfortable lying on your stomach, switch to the hands and knees position found in the **THIRD TRIMESTER WORKOUT** or place a small pillow or towel under your **hip bones and pubic bone**.

TRANSITION:

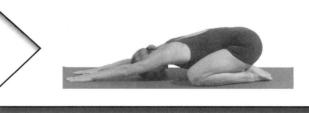

Bend your knees and push back toward your heels with your knees slightly apart and your hands reaching for your ankles. Your forehead is on the floor.

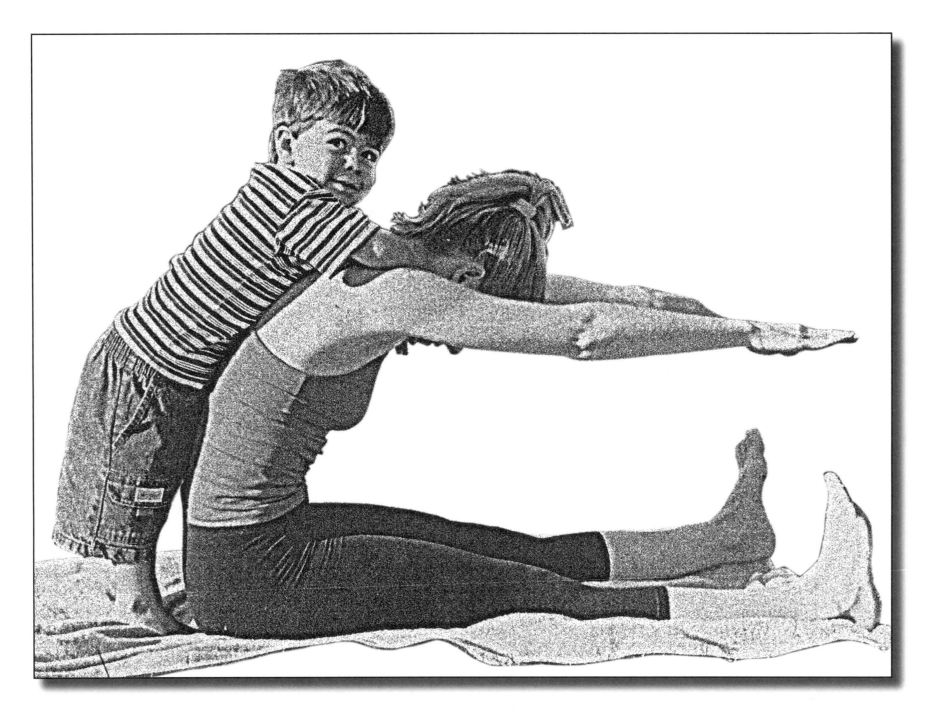

Child's Pose/A Little Piece of Heaven

What is needed:

NOTES:

GOAL: To relax the muscles of your back.

PRENATAL BENEFITS: When you are pregnant, you can expect your back is going to ache from time to time. This exercise is fantastic for releasing those tight muscles.

POSITION:

SIT back on your heels with your forehead on the floor in front of you. Your feet are together but your knees are slightly apart. Your arms are on the floor in front of you.

EXECUTION:

SIMPLY relax. Allow your back muscles to stretch and open up. This is a great position to practice your **BREATHING.**

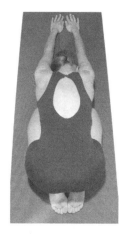

Helpful Hints:

Imagine your back is your stomach, let it rise and fall.

SIT WITH YOUR LEGS UNCROSSED.

MODIFICATION:

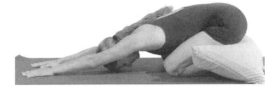

Place a pillow behind your knees if you have knee discomfort.

TRANSITION:

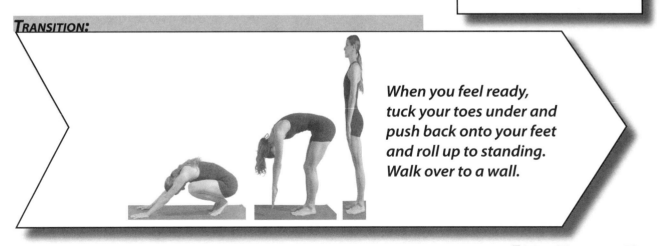

When you feel ready, tuck your toes under and push back onto your feet and roll up to standing. Walk over to a wall.

Round Down With Push Up

What is needed:

NOTES:

_____

_____

_____

_____

_____

_____

GOAL: To gain upper body strength while stretching your back and legs.

PRENATAL BENEFITS: Rolling down and up against the wall allows you to feel each vertebra to make sure that your lower spine is not overly arched. **ROUND DOWN** allows you to get a great stretch in the muscles of your back and legs.

POSITION:

STAND with your back against the wall, legs parallel and hip width apart. Feet are about six inches away from the wall. You are in **neutral pelvis**. Your lower back may not touch but **imprint** the rest of your spine.

EXECUTION:

INHALE as you **imprint** pressing your back into the wall. Raise your arms over your head while keeping your shoulders and ribs down.

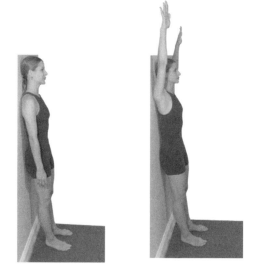

EXHALE and peel your back off the wall one **vertebra** at a time, as you roll all the way down. Every **vertebra** in your spine has to touch the wall before it peels off. Pull the abdominal muscles toward your baby and go through a **pelvic tilt**. Finish with your hands on the floor. Your legs may be bent.

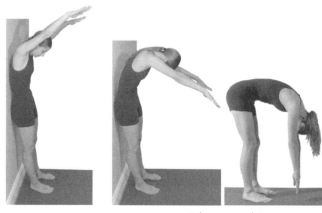

Helpful Hints:

Imagine you are doing a standing ROLL UP against the wall.

Pilates and Pregnancy

EXECUTION (CONTINUED):

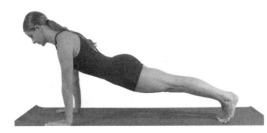

INHALE and walk your hands out so that your body is in a **push-up** position.

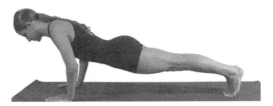

KEEPING your arms tight against your body, do three **tricep** push-ups. Exhale as your arms bend; inhale as they straighten.

This is one push-up.

Do three push-ups.

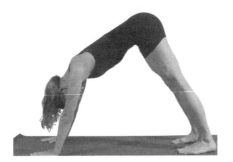

EXHALE to lift your hips high while lowering your heels to give your legs a brief stretch.

If your lower back arches and you feel strain in your **powerhouse,** stop. Do the modification.

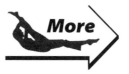
More

ROUND all the way up.

INHALE to walk your hands back to your feet.

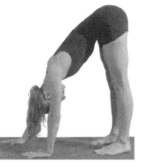

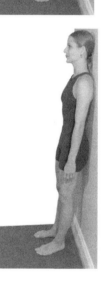

EXHALE and place your buttocks against the wall.

AGAIN, try to get each **vertebra** to touch the wall. Straighten your legs as you uncurl.

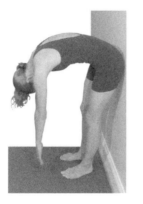

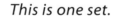

This is one set.

Do three sets with three push-ups in each set.

MODIFICATION:

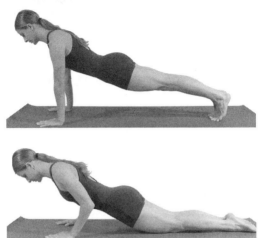

If the push-up is too difficult to do with your belly lifted and back straight, try just holding the push up position for a few breaths. If you are still feeling this in your back, a traditional position may be a future goal. For now, let your knees touch the floor.

For your review:

Did you need to skip this exercise today?

_____

_____

How did this exercise feel today?

_____

_____

Did you need to modify anything?

_____

_____

Did your baby react more or less today?

_____

_____

TRANSITION:

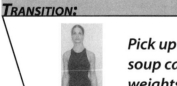

Pick up the soup cans or weights and return your back to the wall.

Curls

What is needed:

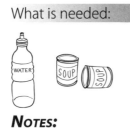

NOTES:

_____

_____

_____

_____

_____

GOAL: To build upper body strength and leg stamina.

PRENATAL BENEFITS: Your upper body strength will help you carry your baby after birth. Sitting in an invisible chair against the wall helps build stamina.

POSITION:

START with your back against the wall with your legs parallel and **hip-width apart**. Your feet are about a foot away from the wall.

INHALE as you slide your back down the wall until your legs are at a ninety-degree angle or greater. Watch your leg alignment. Keep your knees over the toes and in line with your feet.

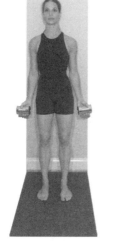
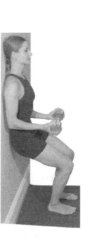

EXECUTION:

Do four **BICEP CURLS.**

EXHALE as you curl your arms up.

INHALE as you lower your arms. End on an inhale.

Helpful Hints:

Keep your **navel-to-spine.** Keep your spine in contact with the wall.

Focus straight ahead.

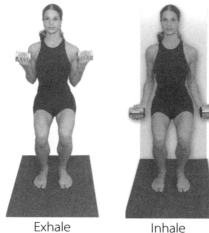

Exhale   Inhale

EXHALE to lift your arms shoulder height and open them against the wall.

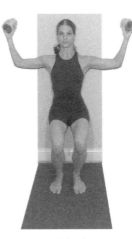

Exhale

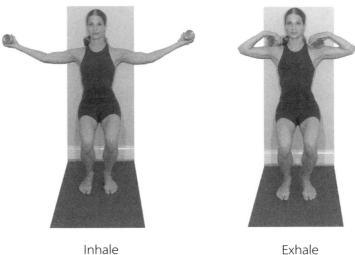

Inhale   Exhale

Do four **BICEP CURLS** with your arms against the wall.

INHALE as you extend your forearms.

EXHALE as you curl them in. Finish on an exhale.

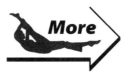

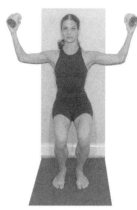

Inhale

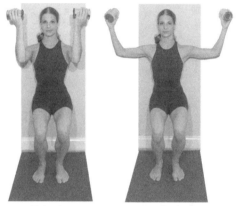

Exhale   Inhale

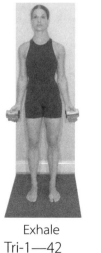

Exhale

INHALE and open your arms to a ninety-degree angle against the wall.

EXHALE and bring them in front of your shoulders with your triceps parallel to the floor.

INHALE as your return them to the wall.

REPEAT opening and closing your arms four times. Finish on an inhale with your arms against the wall.

EXHALE as you straighten your legs and lower your arms. Take a brief rest.

This is one set.

Do two sets of all three curls.

MODIFICATION:

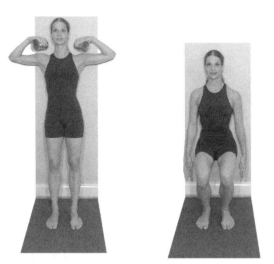

You can choose to only do the **CURLS** without bending your knees or you can sit in an invisible chair without the weights.

TRANSITION:

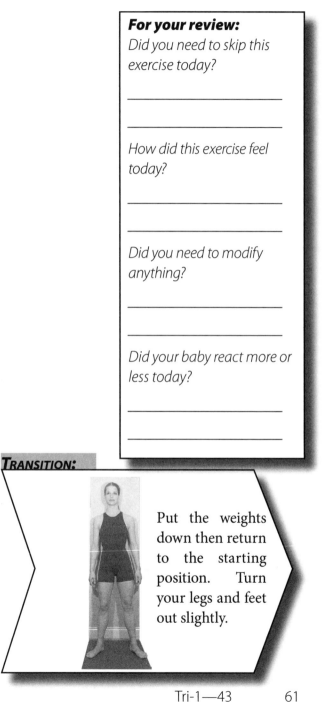

Put the weights down then return to the starting position. Turn your legs and feet out slightly.

Squat

What is needed:

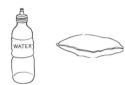

NOTES:

_____

_____

_____

_____

_____

_____

GOAL: To stretch your lower back, inner thigh and calves.

PRENATAL BENEFITS: The leg stamina gained from this exercise is a terrific way to build toward squatting in labor. Squatting during labor utilizes gravity to help speed up the birthing process.

POSITION:

STAND with your back against the wall. Your legs are about hip-width apart. Your feet and legs are slightly turned out. Your feet are six-to-eight inches from the wall.

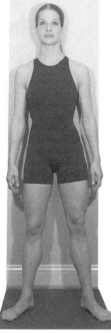

EXECUTION:

SLIDE all the way down to the floor, keeping your heels on the floor and your knees over your feet. Imprint your back against the wall.

PRACTICE your breathing.

ALLOW your inner thighs and pelvis to release and open.

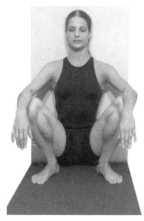

Helpful Hints:

Do not roll in on your feet.

Keep your torso lifted out of your legs.

Pilates and Pregnancy

EAT SEVERAL SMALL MEALS A DAY RATHER THAN THREE BIG ONES.

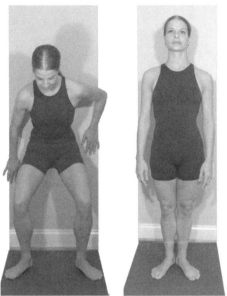

ON your own time, walk your hands back up the wall to help you straighten your legs and come to standing.

Step away from the wall with your feet in a **Pilates V** and stack your vertebrae one on top of the other. Keep your abdominal muscles reaching upward that your torso is well supported.

Try to remember this posture for the rest of the day.

MODIFICATION:

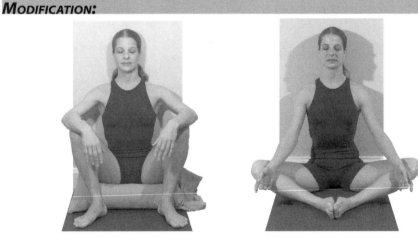

If you have knee problems, support yourself on a pillow or sit on the floor with your back against the wall and the bottom of your feet together. Don't force your legs. Allow gravity to open your thighs.

WEIGHT AT THE BEGINNING OF THE 1ST TRIMESTER: _____

WEIGHT AT THE END OF THE 1ST TRIMESTER: _____

BLOOD PRESSURE AT THE BEGINNING OF THE 1ST TRIMESTER: _____

BLOOD PRESSURE AT THE END OF THE 1ST TRIMESTER: _____

TEST/RESULTS: _____

HOW DOES YOUR BODY FEEL? _____ *BACK PAIN?* _____ *SCIATICA?* _____ *TIGHTNESS?* _____

DID ANY EXERCISES FEEL ESPECIALLY GOOD? _____ *HOW?* _____

DID YOU AVOID OR MODIFY ANY EXERCISES? _____ *WHY?* _____

HOW MANY DAYS PER WEEK DID YOU DO PILATES AND PREGNANCY? _____

HOW MANY DAYS PER WEEK DID YOU DO LIGHT CARDIO? _____

DATE: _____

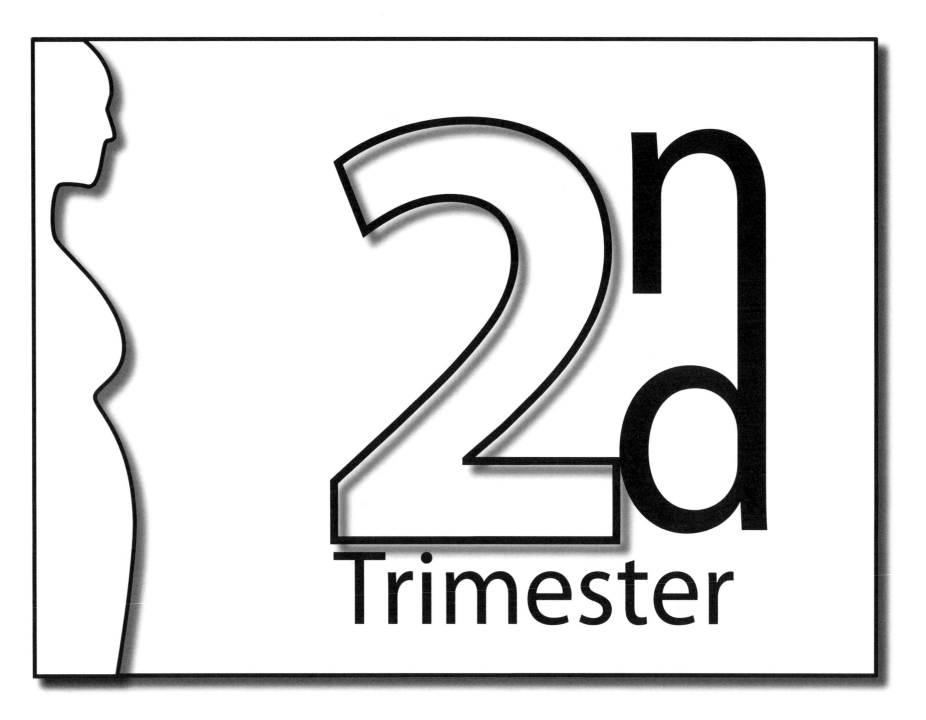

2nd Trimester

Second Trimester Workout

You will need:

After the fourth month, the weight of your growing uterus can put too much pressure on the **vena cava** (a major vein supplying blood to both you and your baby) while you are lying on your back. All the exercises have been modified for use on an incline. If you feel nauseous at any time, roll onto your left side. This is the position for the greatest freedom of blood flow. Even if you do not get nauseous while lying on your back, many medical professionals feel you may still be impeding blood flow. Therefore, I recommend beginning this workout after your fourth month even if you still feel comfortable on your back.

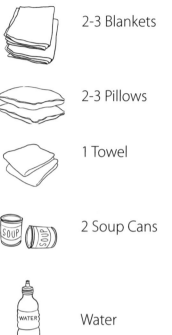

2-3 Blankets

2-3 Pillows

1 Towel

2 Soup Cans

Water

During this trimester, emphasis is beginning to shift from intense abdominal work to leg strength, relaxation and controlled flexibility. The incline transfers some of the burden of stability to your legs and buttocks, which will need to be toned to carry the added weight of pregnancy. Depending on the size of your belly, you may need to take your legs a little wider when a **hip-width** position is called for. You will need to adjust your leg position periodically to make room for your growing belly. You will also find that the abdominal areas targeted in this series of exercises will move higher to the upper **rectus** and **external obliques**. However, the deep **pelvic floor** is also being toned. Even though many of the exercises in this trimester are the same ones described in the previous chapter, they will look and feel different because of the modified use of an incline and because of your changing physique.

The exercises in this section are being demonstrated by Dana, who is twenty-five weeks pregnant with her second baby.

How To Build An Incline

What is needed:

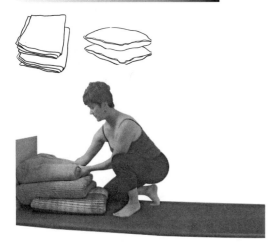

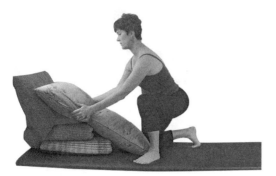

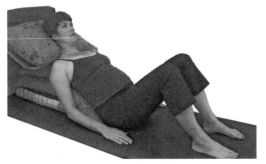

FOLD your blankets into rectangles and stack them on top of each other like stairs. Lean your pillows against the blankets. Adjust them until you are comfortable with the degree of incline. The incline must be placed against something stationary.

Breathing

What is needed:

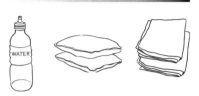

NOTES:

_____

_____

_____

GOAL: To learn to breath into your **ribcage** and lower back while not allowing your belly to rise and fall. This will increase the space between your ribs to allow for maximum air intake. The more you practice the **PILATES BREATHING** the greater your lung capacity will be.

PRENATAL BENEFITS: Remember, your internal organs are starting to push into your **ribcage**, so help make room for them by increasing the space between your ribs. This will allow more room for your lungs to fully expand. Pregnancy hormones already do some of the work for you by increasing the space between your ribs.

POSITION:

LIE on incline. Feet flat, knees bent. Imprint your spine into the incline.

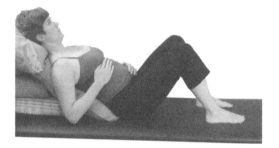

Helpful Hints:

Remember, **BREATHING** expands your **ribcage** sideways and back.

Since it is the foundation for all the movement and is so difficult to master, I recommend working on **BREATHING** every day. You will also find it meditative and relaxing to practice conscious **breathing.**

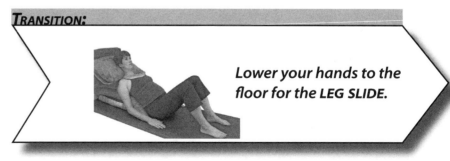

EXECUTION:

INHALE deeply into your lower back while letting your ribcage expand sideways and back.

EXHALE and send your ribs down toward your hips.

INHALE through your nose exhale out of your mouth.

Take at least ten breaths.

For your review:

Did you need to skip this exercise today?

_____

_____

How did this exercise feel today?

_____

_____

Did you need to modify anything?

_____

_____

Did your baby react more or less today?

_____

_____

TRANSITION:

Lower your hands to the floor for the LEG SLIDE.

Leg Slides

What is needed:

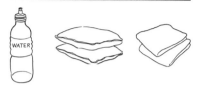

NOTES:

_____

_____

_____

_____

_____

_____

GOAL: To lengthen your leg muscles.

PRENATAL BENEFITS: **Relaxin** loosens the joints during pregnancy. This exercise helps train your body to move with control while lengthening your leg muscles.

POSITION:

LIE on your back, legs bent **hip-width apart.** Palms are lightly pressing the floor at your sides. **Pelvis** is in neutral and shoulders are wide and relaxed.

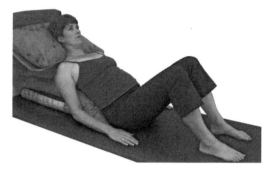

EXECUTION:

INHALE and flex your right foot. Slide it along the floor until your leg is straight. Make sure your **powerhouse** are drawn in and up to prevent your **pelvis** from moving and your back from arching.

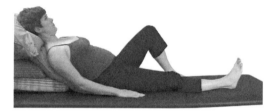

Helpful Hints:

To understand the role of the **hamstring** in this exercise, imagine how you would pick up a heavy object. You wouldn't try to lift it from the top; you would pick it up from underneath. The same is true for your leg. The underneath muscle controls the leg coming back in.

Place your hands on your hips occasionally to make sure your hips stay level and don't move.

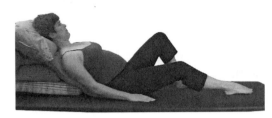

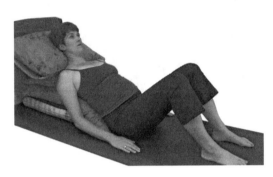

EXHALE as you point your foot and bring your leg back to the starting position. Use your **powerhouse** and your **hamstring** to do this. Feel weight in your opposite foot and hip.

Repeat using your left leg.

This is one set.

Do three sets.

For your review:

Did you need to skip this exercise today?

_____

_____

How did this exercise feel today?

_____

_____

Did you need to modify anything?

_____

_____

Did your baby react more or less today?

_____

_____

TRANSITION:

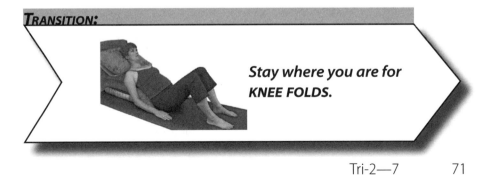

Stay where you are for KNEE FOLDS.

Knee Folds

1 2 3 4 5

What is needed:

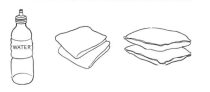

NOTES:

_____

_____

_____

_____

_____

GOAL: To train your **powerhouse** to initiate all movement so that you can move with control and ease. The stronger your torso, the lighter your limbs will feel.

PRENATAL BENEFITS: The focus on preventing your back from arching further is an imperative strengthening exercise during pregnancy. It will limit further back strains. Hopefully this kind of abdominal awareness will become second nature in everyday activities.

POSITION:

LIE on the incline with your legs bent, feet flat on the floor slightly wider than **hip-width apart**.

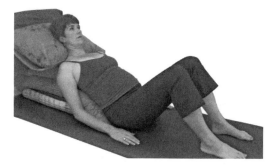

EXECUTION:

EXHALE to draw your right leg into a ninety-degree angle. Keep your foot relaxed so that you don't activate the front of your thigh (**quadriceps**) and calf muscle. Make sure your **pelvis** is in **neutral**. Your stomach is pulled in and up to prevent your back from arching.

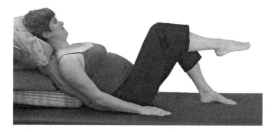

Helpful Hints:

The **powerhouse** actually initiates your leg movement. Put weight on your standing foot to help that hip stay on the same plane as your working hip.

Alternate resting one hand on your hip to make sure your opposite hip stays still when your leg moves.

SHEA BUTTER IS GREAT ON ITCHY SKIN.

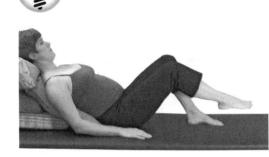

INHALE as you lower your leg. Again, make sure your stomach doesn't stick out as you lower your leg. Your abdominal muscles are actively moving in and up as your leg moves.

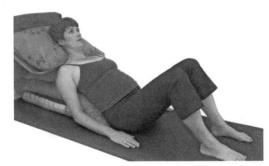

Repeat using your left leg.

This is one set.

Do three sets.

Stop if you feel your abdominal muscles push out or your back arch. Try again when you are stronger.

For your review:

Did you need to skip this exercise today?

_____

_____

How did this exercise feel today?

_____

_____

Did you need to modify anything?

_____

_____

Did your baby react more or less today?

_____

_____

TRANSITION:

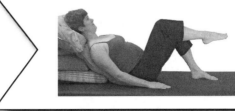

After your left leg lowers in the third set, KNEE FOLD the right leg one more time and leave it in chair position.

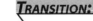

The Hundred

What is needed:

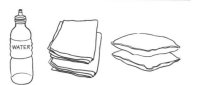

NOTES:

GOAL: To increase circulation while toning your **powerhouse.**

PRENATAL BENEFITS: Because you are lying on an incline, and your torso is close to your extended leg, your inner thigh gets a greater workout. The buttocks and **hamstring** of your standing leg also work harder to maintain your body on the incline. This exercise not only tones your abdominal muscles and inner thigh, it gets your blood circulating. Blood volume almost doubles during pregnancy, so it is important to keep it circulating well to prevent it from pooling in your legs, which can contribute to edema and varicose veins.

POSITION:

LIE on the incline, legs bent and together, feet flat on the floor.

INHALE and lift your head and shoulders off the incline, curving your upper back like a light post. Keep your neck relaxed and in a long curve. Reach your arms off the floor a few inches.

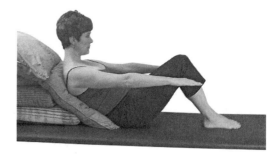

EXHALE to extend your right leg, turned out at a forty-five-degree angle. Your inner thighs stay together. Keep your right foot relaxed. Your left foot is flat on the floor. Take your focus to your extended knee.

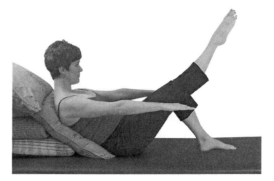

Helpful Hints:

Just because you are pregnant doesn't mean your abdominal muscles become inactive.

Imagine that you are wearing a corset that is laced up in front.

HORMONES AND UTERINE PRESSURE ON YOUR BLADDER CAUSE YOU TO URINATE MORE FREQUENTLY.

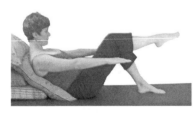

EXECUTION:

PUMP your arms up and down while slowly inhaling for five counts and slowly exhaling for five counts.

This is one set.

Do five sets with your right leg extended.

WITHOUT lowering your upper back, alternate legs. To switch legs, turn your right leg parallel, bend and lower your foot to the ground. Extend your left leg, turned out while keeping your inner thighs connected.

Do five more sets with your left leg extended.

For your review:

Did you need to skip this exercise today?

_____

_____

How did this exercise feel today?

_____

_____

Did you need to modify anything?

_____

_____

Did your baby react more or less today?

_____

_____

MODIFICATION:

Lying on an incline will actually make it more difficult to keep your leg between a forty-five-degree and a ninety-degree angle. If you are having difficulty in this position, you can keep the working leg bent in **chair position** or keep both feet on the floor.

TRANSITION:

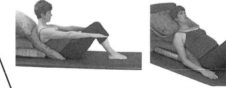

Parallel your left leg and lower your foot to the floor. Your legs will end up together. Return your upper back and arms to the floor. Bring your legs hip-width apart. Make sure your feet are truly parallel with your knees in line with your feet.

Bridging

What is needed:

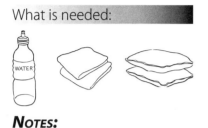

NOTES:

_____

_____

_____

_____

GOAL: To increase mobility in your back and pelvis. To stretch your hip flexors and quadriceps while toning your inner thighs, buttocks and hamstrings.

PRENATAL BENEFITS: Bridging helps stretch the front of your thighs and hips as well as your spine. Tucking your pelvis helps to relieve the exaggerated arch in your lower back that tends to occur during pregnancy.

POSITION:

LIE on the incline. Your legs are bent, slightly wider than **hip-width apart.** Your hands are at your sides, palms down. Keep your shoulders wide and your neck relaxed.

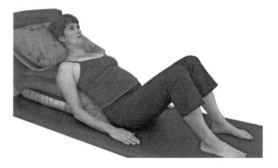

EXECUTION:

INHALE as you tilt your **pubic bone** up towards your belly button.

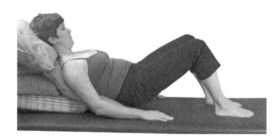

Helpful Hints:

Try to send your energy toward your knees to really lengthen your back as you roll down.

It is tempting to push up all at once with the thighs and bypass the stomach. Resist this temptation!

EXHALE and press your feet into the ground while continuing to peel each **vertebra** off the floor one at a time by first melting the front of your body toward the incline. Only come up about two-thirds of the way to prevent your neck and shoulders from compressing. Try to roll up sequentially rather than pressing up all at once.

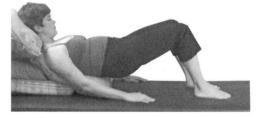

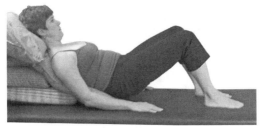

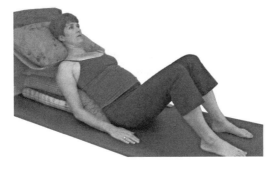

INHALE as you start rolling down by softening your **sternum** and sending your ribs toward your hips. Watch your leg alignment. Pull your inner thighs toward each other to prevent your legs from opening.

EXHALE and continue to roll down. Don't skip the deep **pelvic tilt** at the bottom that allows your lower back to sink into the incline.

RETURN to a **neutral pelvis**.

This is one set.

Do four sets.

For your review:

Did you need to skip this exercise today?

_____

_____

How did this exercise feel today?

_____

_____

Did you need to modify anything?

_____

_____

Did your baby react more or less today?

_____

_____

TRANSITION:

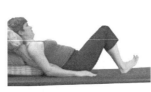

Close your legs; flex your feet and slide them all the way down. Inhale your arms up over your shoulders. Exhale moving your arms over your head, without letting your ribs pop open or your hands touch the incline.

Roll Up

What is needed:

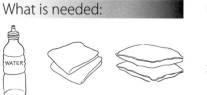

NOTES:

_____

_____

_____

_____

Helpful Hints:

Being on an incline makes it possible for more women to do this exercise with the traditionally straight legs since you are already part way up to begin with.

Let your legs and arms reach forward as your belly and back pull behind you. This oppositional stretch will help ground you.

GOAL: To stretch your back and your legs while working your entire **powerhouse.**

PRENATAL BENEFITS: Doing **ROLL UP** on an incline takes some of the pressure off the abdominal muscles. They are still being worked, but now you can concentrate on the benefits of stretching your back and your legs.

POSITION:

LIE on your incline with your legs together and extended along the floor, feet flexed. Arms are extended over your head without touching the incline. Keep your ribs down so that your back stays in contact with the incline.

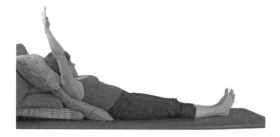

EXECUTION:

INHALE and curl your head and shoulders off the incline keeping your head between your arms,.

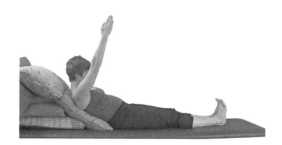

EXHALE and continue to roll up one **vertebra** at a time. Let your abdominal muscles hug your baby rather than pulling away from her. Try to round your back as much as possible.

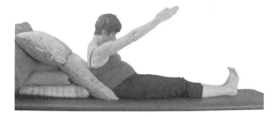

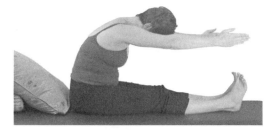

Continue to a seated position with your body in a C shaped curve. Leave room for your belly. Arms are parallel to the floor. Keep your shoulders down. Your head is still between your arms and the back of your neck long.

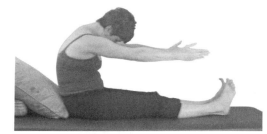

Inhale as you tuck your **pelvis** under and begin to roll down.

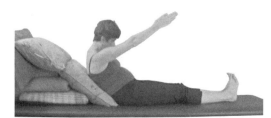

Exhale while continuing your descent. Make sure each part of your back touches the incline. Try to keep your arms in line with your ears. Return to the starting position.

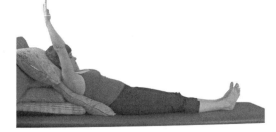

This is one set.

Do six sets.

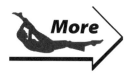

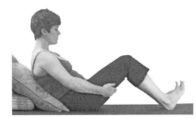

If you are still uncomfortable rolling up with your legs straight, keep your feet flexed and bend your legs.

PLACE your hands behind your thighs to help you pull your back into a C curve.

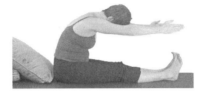

EXTEND your legs and come to the same seated position described in ROLL UP.

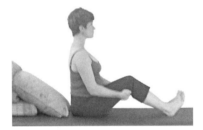

BEND your knees as you SIT TALL.

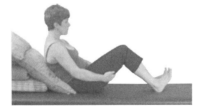

HOLD on to your legs to roll back down.

For your review:

Did you need to skip this exercise today?

_____

_____

How did this exercise feel today?

_____

_____

Did you need to modify anything?

_____

_____

Did your baby react more or less today?

_____

_____

TRANSITION:

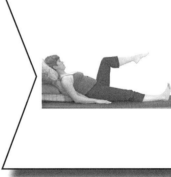

After the last set, lower your arms to your sides. Point your right foot, bend your leg and float it to chair position. Remember to use the same LEG SLIDE and KNEE FOLD skills you already worked on.

THOUGHTS AND FEELINGS

Date: _____

This time in my pregnancy has been... _____

_____

_____

_____

_____

I feel good about my body because... _____

_____

_____

_____

_____

I am anxious about... _____

_____

_____

_____

Leg Circles

What is needed:

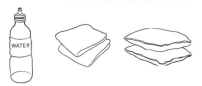

NOTES:

_____

_____

_____

GOAL: To increase circulation and mobility of your leg and hip joint while strengthening your **powerhouse.**

PRENATAL BENEFITS: Lying on an incline makes this a harder workout for your inner thigh. Elevating your leg will stimulate your circulation and reduce swelling.

POSITION:

LIE on the incline with your left leg extended along the floor, foot flexed. Your right leg is turned out and lengthened toward the ceiling, with your foot relaxed. Keep your **pelvis** in **neutral.** Make sure your neck and shoulders are relaxed and open.

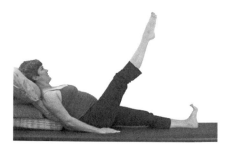

Helpful Hints:

Press your palms into the floor and imagine that you are standing on your extended leg.

Remember, this is an abdominal exercise so initiate the movement from your **powerhouse.**

Keep your hips even and your back against the incline.

EXECUTION:

WHILE keeping your body completely still by engaging your **powerhouse**, isolate your leg and make circles. (Cross the center of your body, bring it down slightly, open it slightly past your hip and return it to the starting position. Pause at the top.)

INHALE for half the circle. Exhale for half and pause at the top.

This completes one circle.

Make five circles in one direction.

Reverse the direction for five circles.

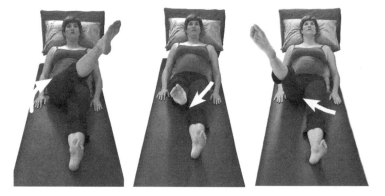

Cross the center of your body.

Bring your leg down slowly.

Open just past your hips and return to the starting position.

Pause at the top.

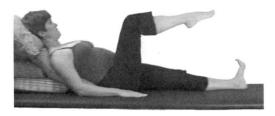

SWITCH legs:

TURN your right leg parallel, bend it and lower it to the ground.

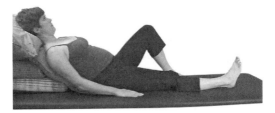

FLEX your left foot and elongate your leg. Point your left foot and bend your left leg in.

Go through **chair position** to extend your left leg turned out to the ceiling.

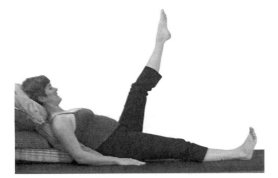

MAKE five circles in both directions with your left leg.

❗ Be careful not to make your circle larger than it was last trimester. You have less abdominal strength to draw from now.

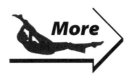 **More** ➤

MODIFICATION:

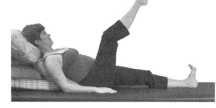

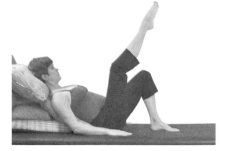

Modifications: If your tailbone starts tucking under bend your working leg or bend your bottom leg and put your foot flat on the floor.

For your review:

Did you need to skip this exercise today?

_____

_____

How did this exercise feel today?

_____

_____

Did you need to modify anything?

_____

_____

Did your baby react more or less today?

_____

_____

TRANSITION:

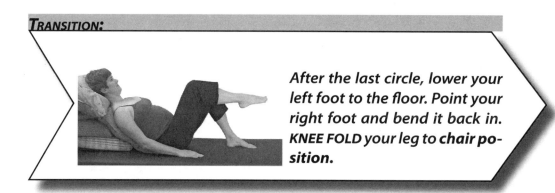

After the last circle, lower your left foot to the floor. Point your right foot and bend it back in. KNEE FOLD your leg to chair position.

MY MID-PREGNANCY CHECKLIST

Mid-pregnancy Dental check-up: Date: _____ Notes: _____

_____

My Baby is Registered at: _____

Plan for [solicit, recruit, sign-up] friends and family who will help you for a few days after the baby is born.

   Cook: _____

   Clean: _____

   Laundry: _____

   Groceries: _____

   Caring for older siblings (feed, take to school/other activities): _____

_____

Make sure someone will watch any older children when you go into labor:

Name: _____ Home Phone:_____ Cell: _____

Register for Labor Class: Where: _____ When: _____

Stomach Series

What is needed:

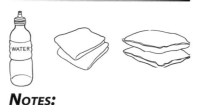

NOTES:

_____

_____

_____

_____

Helpful Hints:

It is more important than ever not to crunch your torso when rounding your upper back. Your belly needs as much room as possible.

Keep your pelvis from tucking by not drawing in your knee too far. Reach your tailbone down in opposition.

The stomach series is designed to target all four abdominal muscle groups. There are five exercises in the series. We will do two of them.

GOAL: To build abdominal strength and stretch your lower back.

PRENATAL BENEFITS: Even though your abdominal muscles are getting a less intense workout, you are building the muscle memory necessary to get you through delivery faster. The leg strength developed will aid in supporting your increasing weight, and building leg stamina will help you through the many positions you may choose to labor in.

Single Leg Stretch

⚠2 ⚠3 ⚠4 ⚠5

POSITION:

LIE on an incline, with your left foot flat on the floor and your right leg in **CHAIR POSITION**. Your right leg is angled more toward your armpit to make room for your belly. Your right hand is on your right ankle and your left hand is on your right knee. Inhale to raise your head and shoulders off the incline so that your torso remains long and your upper back curves up. Keep your **pelvis** in **neutral**.

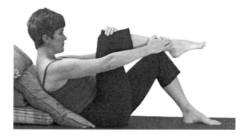

EXECUTION:

EXHALE while gently pulling your right leg in toward your armpit twice. Be sure to leave space between your thigh and your belly.

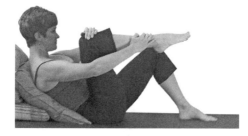

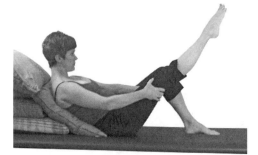

INHALE and extend your right leg at a forty-five-degree angle. It should be the same height as the bent leg. Let your hands slide along your leg as it elongates. Keep your belly drawing in and up.

This is one set.

Do three sets using your right leg.

SWITCH legs and hands without lowering your torso.

Repeat three times using your left leg.

MODIFICATION:

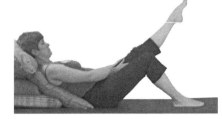

If your neck and shoulders are overly tense, lower your upper back and head to the incline.

TRANSITION:

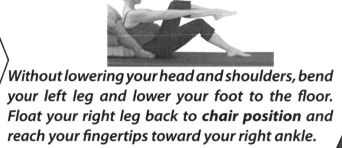

Without lowering your head and shoulders, bend your left leg and lower your foot to the floor. Float your right leg back to chair position and reach your fingertips toward your right ankle.

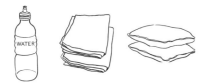

NOTES:

Double Leg Stretch ⚠3 ⚠4 ⚠5

POSITION:

LIE on the incline with your left foot flat on the floor and your right leg in **chair position.** Reach your fingertips to your right ankle while drawing your shoulders back so you don't hunch. Your head and shoulders are off the incline like a curved light post.

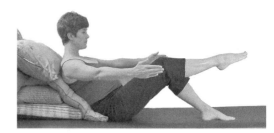

EXECUTION:

INHALE and extend your arms over your head without lowering your torso and extend your right leg turned out from your hip at a forty-five-degree angle. Don't let your arms rest behind you. Focus at your shin.

EXHALE as you turn your leg parallel and bend it back in, letting your arms your arms circle around to the starting position.

This is one set.

Do three sets.

WITHOUT lowering your head and shoulders, switch legs by lowering your right foot to the floor and floating your left leg to **chair position**. Bring your hands to your left ankle. Do not relax your **obliques** while switching sides.

Do three sets with your left leg.

Helpful Hints:

Keep your torso at the same height while extending your leg.

SLEEP WITH A HUMIDIFIER TO ALLEVIATE CONGESTION.

MODIFICATION:

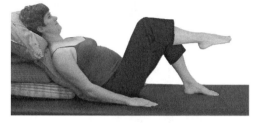

If there is too much strain in your neck, you may lower your head and shoulders to the incline.

For your review:

Did you need to skip this exercise today?

_____

_____

How did this exercise feel today?

_____

_____

Did you need to modify anything?

_____

_____

Did your baby react more or less today?

_____

_____

TRANSITION:

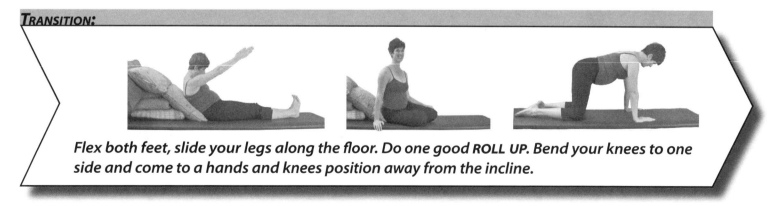

Flex both feet, slide your legs along the floor. Do one good ROLL UP. Bend your knees to one side and come to a hands and knees position away from the incline.

Cat/Side Bend

What is needed:

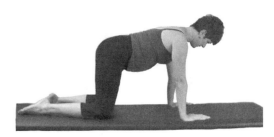

NOTES:

_____

_____

_____

_____

GOAL: To stretch your back.

PRENATAL BENEFITS: This is such a great exercise to get the kinks out of your back. You'll find this very relaxing and soothing as the weight of your belly puts a strain on your back.

POSITION:

COME onto your hands and knees. Make sure your hands are directly under your shoulders and your knees are under your hips. Your back is in **neutral** with your abdominal muscles supporting your baby. Keep your abdominal muscles engaged at all times to prevent your back from sinking under the weight of your belly and overstretching your abdominal muscles.

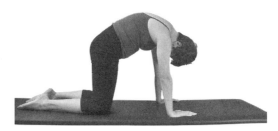

EXECUTION: CAT

EXHALE to round your back, drawing your ribs and belly toward the ceiling while tucking your **pelvis** under. Press into the floor with your palms to really open your upper back. Fully release your head and neck.

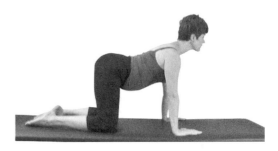

Helpful Hints:

Do **CAT/SIDE BEND** anytime you want relief from backaches.

Keep your shoulders open and down by pressing your palms into the floor.

INHALE to elongate your **spine** so much that it extends into a slight arch. You don't want to sink into your lower back and overstretch your abdominal muscles. Keep the back of your neck long. Try not to collapse into your shoulders.

This is one set of CAT.

Do four sets.

RETURN to the starting position for **SIDE BEND**.

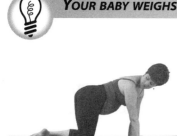

EXECUTION: SIDE BEND

EXHALE. Staying well supported in your belly, bend to the right side as if you were trying to touch your right hip to your right shoulder. Press your palms into the floor to try to keep your **shoulder blades** down and wide.

INHALE. Return to the starting position.
Repeat to the left.

This is one set.

Do four sets.

For your review:

Did you need to skip this exercise today?

_____

_____

How did this exercise feel today?

_____

_____

Did you need to modify anything?

_____

_____

Did your baby react more or less today?

_____

_____

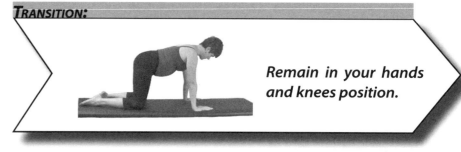

TRANSITION:

Remain in your hands and knees position.

Swimming

What is needed:

WATER

NOTES:

_____

_____

_____

GOAL: To improve your posture and back strength.

PRENATAL BENEFITS: Your back must be strong to counteract the pull of your growing belly. Back strength is as important as abdominal strength in maintaining a healthy back and posture. If you have ever had a back injury, you may have been given a version of SWIMMING by your doctor.

POSITION:

NORMALLY, this exercise is done on your stomach but for the next two trimesters, you are on your hands and knees in the same position as **CAT/SIDE BEND**. It is very important that your belly stays supported. Keep your nose pointing toward the floor.

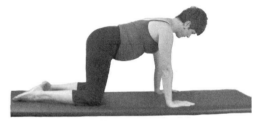

EXECUTION:

INHALE as you slide your right arm forward until it floats up parallel to the floor.

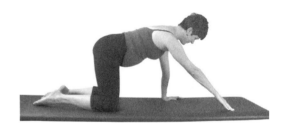

Helpful Hints:

Your shoulder must reach down in opposition to your arm reaching forward.

Lift from the back of your knee and buttocks to keep your leg long and straight.

YOUR arm reaches very far without allowing your shoulder to come with it.

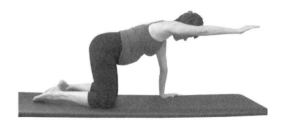

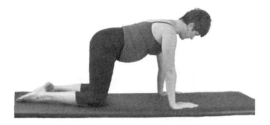

EXHALE and lower your right arm.

SWITCH arms:

INHALE as your left arm lifts and exhale as it lowers.

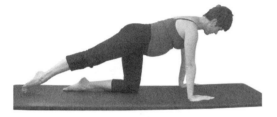

WITHOUT shifting your hips, inhale and reach your right foot back until it floats up parallel to the floor.

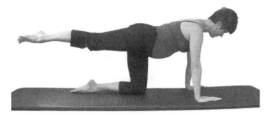

BE careful not to sink into your lower back and shoulders or let your ribs stick out.

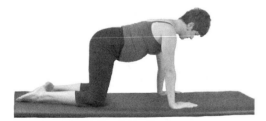

EXHALE to lower your right leg back to the starting position.

SWITCH legs:

INHALE as your left leg lengthens and lifts. Exhale as it lowers.

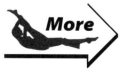

Second Trimester Workout

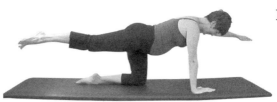

INHALE to reach your left arm and right leg off the floor.

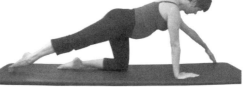

EXHALE as your arm and leg lower.

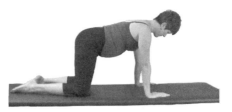

SWITCH sides. Repeat with right arm and left leg.

This is one set.

Do four sets of lifting your arm and leg at the same time.

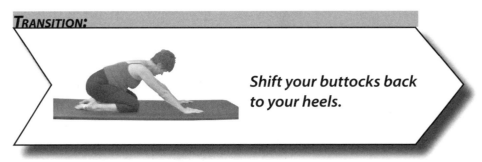

TRANSITION:

Shift your buttocks back to your heels.

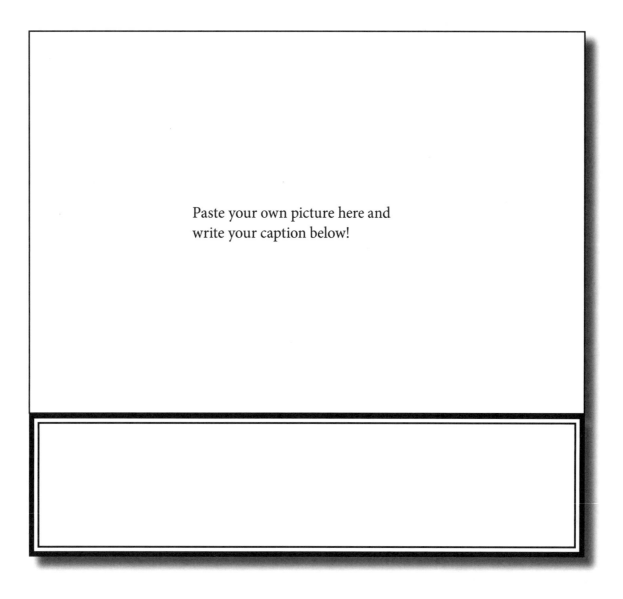

Paste your own picture here and write your caption below!

Child's Pose/A Little Piece of Heaven

What is needed:

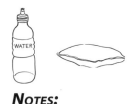

NOTES:

_____

_____

_____

_____

_____

_____

GOAL: To stretch your back.

PRENATAL BENEFITS: To relieve lower back pain associated with pregnancy.

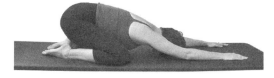

POSITION:

SIT on your heels with your feet together and your knees apart to make room for your belly. Keep your arms on the floor in front of you to support your torso. You will also be stretching your upper back and shoulders.

EXECUTION:

PRACTICE your **BREATHING** by feeling your back rise and fall. Do the hardest thing of all…relax.

Helpful Hints:

Remember, BREATHING expands the ribcage sideways and back, not forward.

BY WEEK 20 YOUR UTERUS WILL BE UP TO YOUR BELLY BUTTON.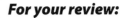

For your review:

Did you need to skip this exercise today?

_____

_____

How did this exercise feel today?

_____

_____

Did you need to modify anything?

_____

_____

Did your baby react more or less today?

_____

_____

MODIFICATION:

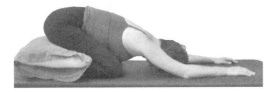

Place a rolled up towel or pillow behind your knees if you experience knee discomfort.

TRANSITION:

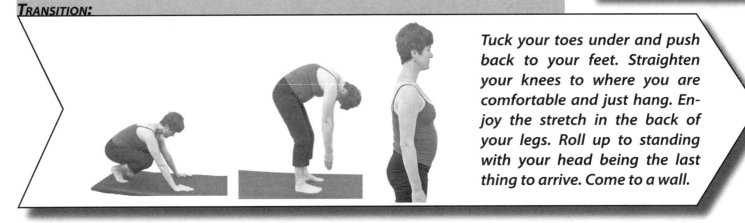

Tuck your toes under and push back to your feet. Straighten your knees to where you are comfortable and just hang. Enjoy the stretch in the back of your legs. Roll up to standing with your head being the last thing to arrive. Come to a wall.

Round Down With Push Up

What is needed:

NOTES:

_____

_____

_____

_____

GOAL: To stretch your back and legs while building arm strength.

PRENATAL BENEFITS: Doing **tricep** pushups in this modified position allows you to get a great upper body and arm workout without undue strain on your back and belly. Rolling down and up against the wall allows you to feel each vertebra to make sure that your lower spine is not overly arched. **ROUND DOWN** allows you to get a great stretch in the muscles of your back and legs.

POSITION:

STAND with your back against the wall and your feet about six inches from the wall. Your legs are parallel and slightly wider than **hip-width apart**. Your **pelvis** is in **neutral**. Imprint your back into the wall as you begin this exercise.

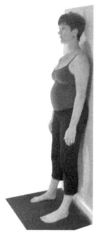

EXECUTION:

INHALE as you bring your arms over your head. Keep your shoulders and ribs down.

EXHALE and peel your back off the wall one **vertebra** at a time, as you roll all the way down. Every **vertebra** in your spine has to touch the wall before it peels off. Pull your abdominal muscles toward your baby and go through a **pelvic tilt.** Finish with your hands on the floor. Your legs may be bent.

Helpful Hints:

Think of this as a standing **ROLL UP.**

Imagine wearing a girdle that supports your baby.

The action of the abdominal muscles has a upward motion much the way they do when you hiccup.

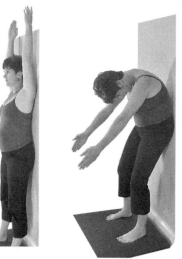

Pilates and Pregnancy

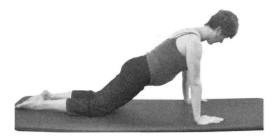

INHALE as you walk your hands out and lower your knees to the floor. Come to a knees-down push up position.

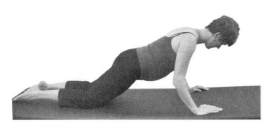

KEEPING your arms close to your body, exhale and lower into a push up. Only go as far as is comfortable.

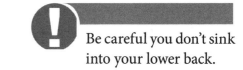

Be careful you don't sink into your lower back.

Be in a **pelvic tilt** to keep your back from arching.

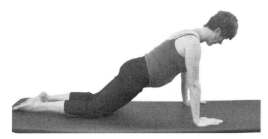

INHALE to straighten your arms. Make sure you support your belly by engaging your **powerhouse.**

This is one push up.

Do three push ups.

Exhale as you push back to CHILD'S POSE.

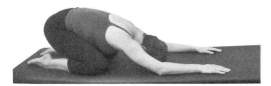

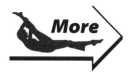

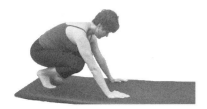

INHALE and tuck your toes under, push onto your feet.

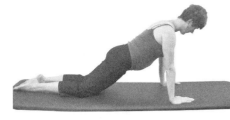

WHILE keeping your knees bent, bring your lower back to the wall.

EXHALE while you straighten your legs and round up, getting each **vertebra** on the wall before returning to the starting position.

This is one set of ROUND DOWN *with push up.*

Do three sets.

For your review:

Did you need to skip this exercise today?

_____

_____

How did this exercise feel today?

_____

_____

Did you need to modify anything?

_____

_____

Did your baby react more or less today?

_____

_____

MODIFICATION:

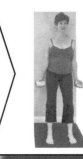

If you feel back strain, go to the push up position, but do not lower your body.

If that is uncomfortable, only round down and up; don't do the push-up.

TRANSITION:

Get two soup cans or light weights and return to the wall.

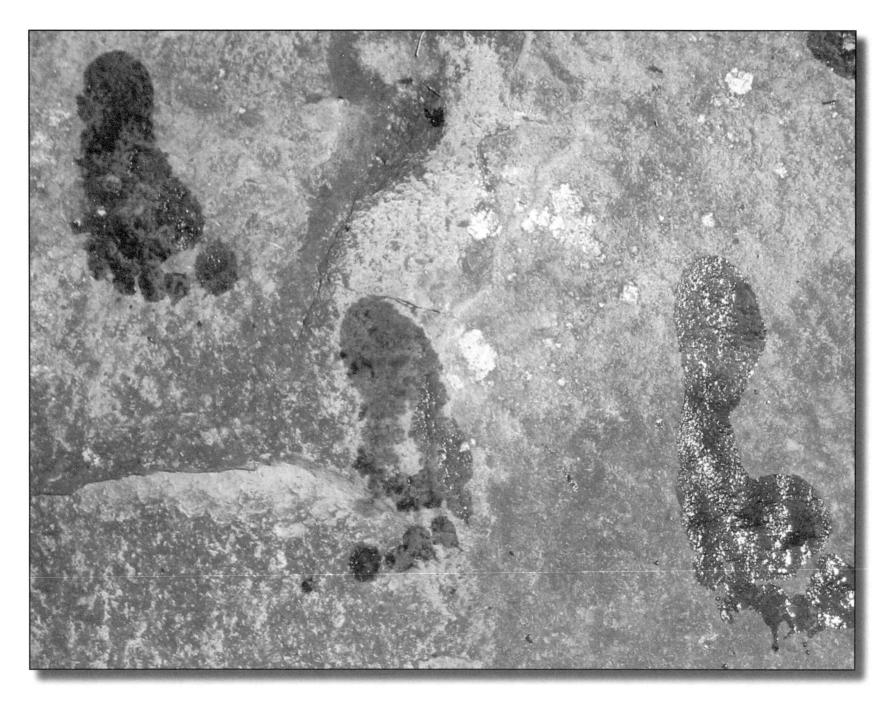

Curls

What is needed:

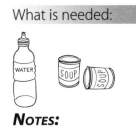

NOTES:

_____

_____

_____

_____

_____

_____

GOAL: To strengthen your upper and lower body.

PRENATAL BENEFITS: In strengthening your arms, shoulders and chest, you are improving your posture while preparing your body to carry your baby. If you would like to squat during labor, this is a great way to build stamina in your legs.

POSITION:

STAND with your back against the wall. Your feet are about a foot away from the wall. Have your legs slightly wider than **hip-width apart.** Keep them parallel. Inhale as you slide down the wall until your legs are at a ninety-degree angle or more. Your knees should not extend beyond your toes. Move your feet forward if they do.

Use the wall to support you. Imprint your back is firmly on the wall.

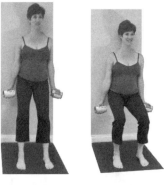

EXECUTION:

Do four **BICEP CURLS.**

EXHALE as you bend your arms. Inhale as you extend them. End on an inhale.

EXHALE to raise your elbows to shoulder height. Rotate your arms so they rest against the wall.

Do four more **BICEP CURLS** in this position.

INHALE to extend your arms against the wall. Exhale as you curl them in. End on an exhale.

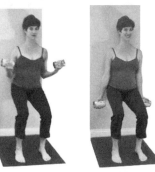

Helpful Hints:

Imprint your spine into the wall and lift your torso up as your legs bend.

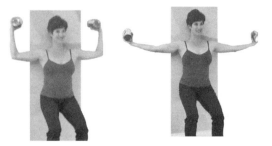

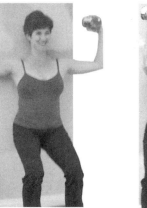 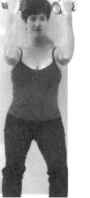

INHALE to open your forearms to a ninety-degree angle. Do four curls in this position with your arms in front.

EXHALE to close your arms in front of your chest.

INHALE to open them back out. Finish on an inhale.

EXHALE to lower your arms and slide back up the wall for a brief rest.

This is one set.

Do two sets of all three CURLS.

For your review:

Did you need to skip this exercise today?

_____

_____

How did this exercise feel today?

_____

_____

Did you need to modify anything?

_____

_____

Did your baby react more or less today?

_____

_____

MODIFICATION:

If you have knee problems, stay standing and only do the curls.

If the weights are too much, you can do this exercise without weights.

TRANSITION:

Put the soup cans down and return to the wall.

Squat

What is needed:

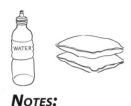

NOTES:

_____

_____

_____

_____

_____

GOAL: To stretch your calves, inner thighs and open your **pelvis.**

PRENATAL BENEFITS: Not only is this position relaxing, but it can help alleviate any tightness in your lower legs and lower back. This is a great position to labor in because it can help your baby descend faster, and it opens the pelvis which helps your baby pass through the birth canal more easily.

POSITION:

Stand with your shoulders, head and lower back against the wall. Your legs can turn out slightly. Your feet will be about six-to-eight inches from the wall. You may need to adjust this so you are comfortable when you **SQUAT.**

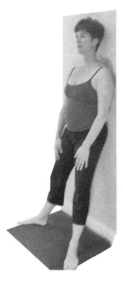

Helpful Hints:

Keep your chest open, shoulders and neck relaxed and your ribcage down.

As you slide down, your entire back will come into contact with the wall.

EXECUTION:

Inhale as you slide all the way down the wall. Keep your heels down. Try not to tuck your **pelvis.** Your belly should stay lifted with your back long and tailbone pointing toward the floor. Practice your **breathing** and just relax. Feel your inner thighs and **pelvis** open and your muscles release. Stay for as long or short a time as you feel comfortable.

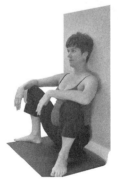

GO FOR A SWIM.

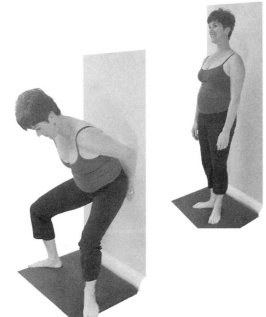

When you are finished, walk your hands up the wall to help you come up to standing.

Step away from the wall with your feet in a **Pilates V**. Try to maintain this posture for the rest of the day.

MODIFICATION:

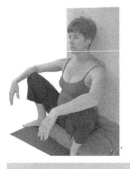

You can sit on a pillow to help support your body. Try to keep your heels down and your whole back and head against the wall.

WEIGHT AT THE BEGINNING OF THE 2ND TRIMESTER: _____

WEIGHT AT THE END OF THE 2ND TRIMESTER: _____

BLOOD PRESSURE AT THE BEGINNING OF THE 2ND TRIMESTER: _____

BLOOD PRESSURE AT THE END OF THE 2ND TRIMESTER: _____

TEST/RESULTS: _____

HOW DOES YOUR BODY FEEL? _____ BACK PAIN? _____ SCIATICA? _____ TIGHTNESS? _____

DID ANY EXERCISES FEEL ESPECIALLY GOOD? _____ HOW? _____

DID YOU AVOID OR MODIFY ANY EXERCISES? _____ WHY? _____

HOW MANY DAYS PER WEEK DID YOU DO PILATES AND PREGNANCY? _____

HOW MANY DAYS PER WEEK DID YOU DO LIGHT CARDIO? _____

DATE: _____

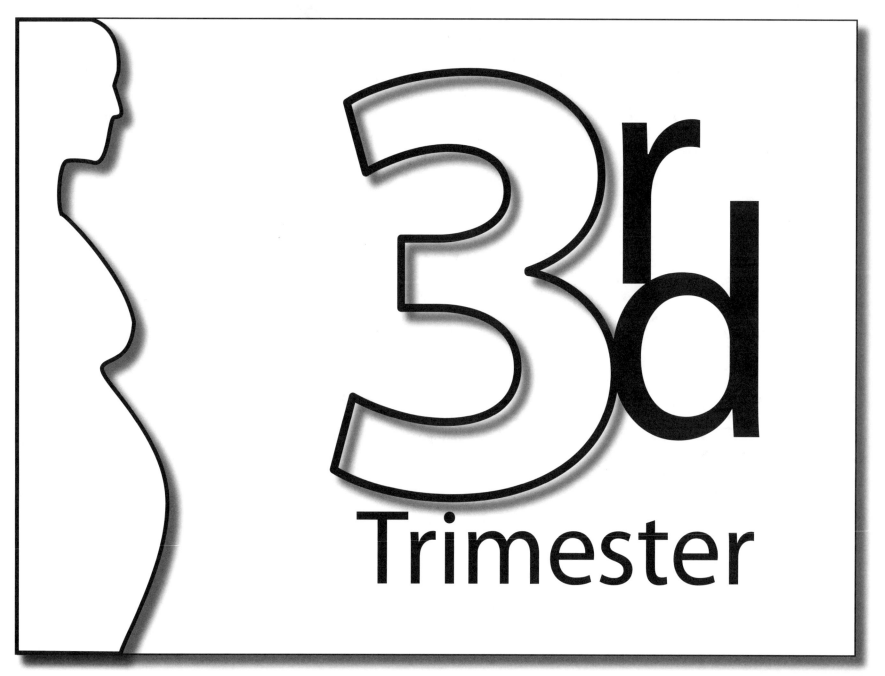

3rd Trimester

Third Trimester Workout

By the time you are in your seventh month, lying on your back, even on an incline, may be uncomfortable and unadvisable. All the exercises for the third trimester have been modified for a sitting, kneeling, standing or side lying position. The larger size of your uterus makes it necessary to take your legs wider than hip-width apart, when called upon. Since balance is also an issue at this stage, you will see that many of the exercises have some sort of a support system. This could be the wall or a heavy piece of furniture.

To help avoid an exercise-induced separation (**diastasys**) of the **rectus muscle** (see TERMS AND TECHNIQUES), intense abdominal work is now replaced by a focus on posture, flexibility, back and arm strength. Take it easy now. You have a lot more weight to carry around, and your body is working over-time to provide nutrients for your baby. This is the trimester where the baby grows the most. You are bound to be more tired. Consult your doctor about continuing your exercise program for the last month.

You will need:

1 Towel

2 Soup Cans

Water

1 Pillow

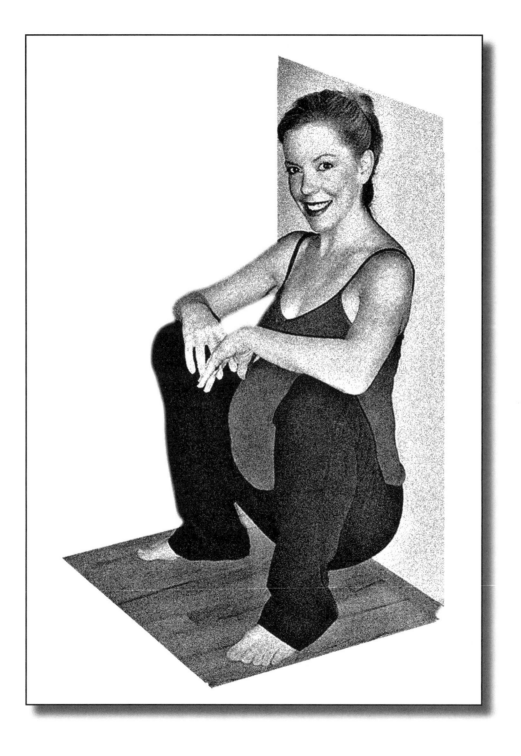

Breathing

What is needed:

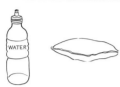

NOTES:

_____

_____

_____

_____

GOAL: To increase the mobility of your ribcage, thus allowing more space for your lungs to expand as the baby grows.

PRENATAL BENEFITS: Now is the time to master this **breathing technique** (if you haven't done so already). Your internal organs are compressed into your **ribcage**, making it difficult to breathe, particularly if you are carrying high. When you go into labor, deep breathing will be the key to pain management. Get good deep breaths that fill the lungs—not just raise the shoulders! Expand the **ribcage** sideways and back to give you power to push during labor. Remember to fully empty your lungs on every exhale. During delivery you will be pushing through an exhalation, so the more lung capacity you have the longer you can sustain a strong push, and the shorter your pushing time will be.

POSITION:

TRY practicing **BREATHING** while sitting. Try to sit tall and relax your legs. Bend your knees slightly if you are having trouble sitting with a straight back.

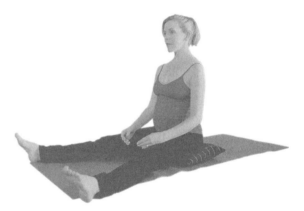

Helpful Hints:

As you inhale, feel your breath go all the way down your lower back.

Keep your neck and shoulders relaxed and open. Let your ribs expand sideways.

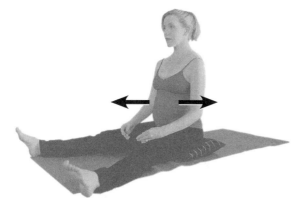

For your review:

Did you need to skip this exercise today?

_____

_____

How did this exercise feel today?

_____

_____

Did you need to modify anything?

_____

_____

Did your baby react more or less today?

_____

_____

EXECUTION:

TRY to feel your ribs move sideways while keeping your shoulders relaxed. Imagine breathing into your lower back and not your chest. Do this several times a day until you've mastered it. Let focusing on your breathing become a relaxation technique.

TAKE at least ten breaths. Inhale through your nose. Exhale through your mouth.

TRANSITION:

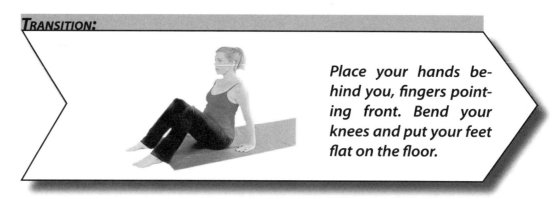

Place your hands behind you, fingers pointing front. Bend your knees and put your feet flat on the floor.

Leg Slides

What is needed:

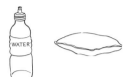

NOTES:

_____

_____

_____

_____

GOAL: To isolate your leg by strengthening your torso.

PRENATAL BENEFITS: It is very tempting to let your posture go at this stage of your pregnancy. Isolating the leg while seated forces you to incorporate back strength to stay lifted and tall in the torso.

POSITION:

SIT on the floor and place your hands behind you with your fingers pointing forward. Your legs are bent, slightly wider than hip width apart. Your back is in **neutral,** so try not to let your **pelvis** tuck under. Feet are flat on the floor.

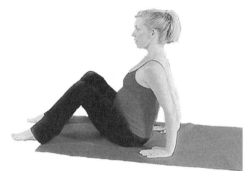

EXECUTION:

INHALE and flex your right foot to slide it along the floor until your leg is straight and very long.

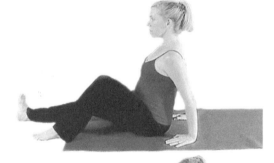

EXHALE as you point your foot, drawing your leg back home. Grow taller in the spine, using the back of your leg and your **powerhouse** to draw your leg in.

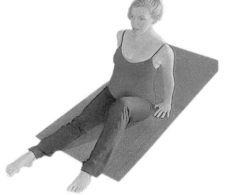

Helpful Hints:

Press into your hands to keep your back long and your shoulders down.

TREAT YOURSELF TO A PRENATAL MASSAGE.

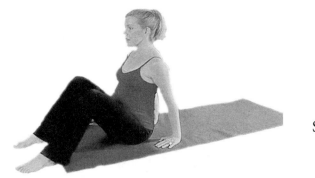

SWITCH legs:

INHALE as you lengthen your left leg. Exhale as you bend it back in.

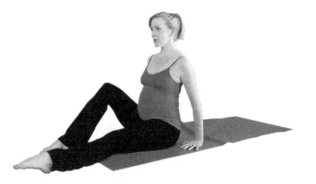

This is one set.

Do three sets.

MODIFICATION:

Sit on a pillow if your **hamstrings** and back are tight. You can also sit against a wall for added support.

TRANSITION:

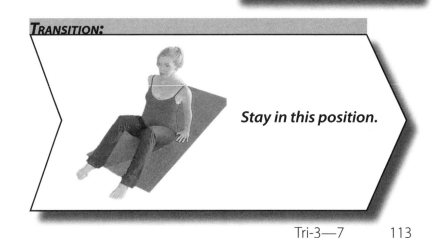

Stay in this position.

Bridging

△1 △2 △3 △4 △5

What is needed:

[water bottle icon] WATER

NOTES:

_____

_____

_____

Helpful Hints:

Imagine that your **pubic bone** is the first to arrive on the way up and last to arrive as you roll down.

Press into your hands to keep your shoulder blades down.

Kegeling will help you engage your deep abdominal muscles.

GOAL: To stretch your back and **hip flexors** while building arm and **hamstring** strength.

PRENATAL BENEFITS: Poor pregnancy posture affects the front of your body as well as your back. This modified exercise helps gently stretch and tone your entire body.

POSITION:

SIT tall with your legs bent, feet slightly wider than hip-width apart. Your hands are behind you, fingertips facing front.

EXECUTION:

BENDING your arms, inhale and rock back into a pelvic tilt.

EXHALE as you continue to roll up to a table top position with your knees over your feet and your shoulders over your hands.

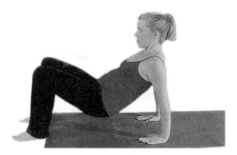

INHALE as you soften your **sternum** and roll down.

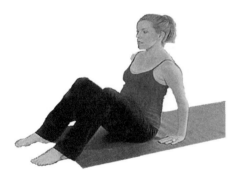

SHIFT your weight back and bend your arms to bring your buttocks back to the starting position.

This is one set.

Do four sets.

TRANSITION:

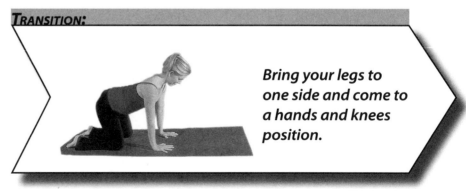

Bring your legs to one side and come to a hands and knees position.

Knee Folds

What is needed:

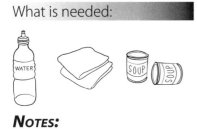

NOTES:

GOAL: To stretch your back and create torso length while engaging the **pelvic floor, transversus** and **oblique** muscles.

PRENATAL BENEFITS: You will be **Kegeling** to initiate movement in this exercise. Getting used to the sensation doing a **Kegel** will help you locate your **transversus.** Learning to **Kegel** is important for vaginal tightness, bladder control and support of internal organs. Keeping your back in **neutral** while bending your leg in will help stretch your lower back. Finding these deep abdominal and back muscles will help improve posture.

Helpful Hints:

Fight the urge to round your back by thinking of reaching your **tailbone** away from your shoulders.

Kegel as you draw your leg in, to help find the deep lower abdominal muscles needed.

Imagine your abdominal wall is a sling for your baby, that ties in the center of your back.

Just because you are focusing on the lower body doesn't mean the upper body is inactive.

POSITION:

COME onto your hands and knees with your knees directly under your hips and your hands directly under your shoulders. Keep your back in **neutral** with your belly well supported. Without moving your hands, pull your palms backward pressing against the floor to keep your shoulders down and wide.

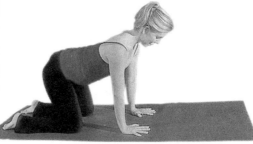

EXECUTION:

WITHOUT rounding your back, exhale and draw your right knee toward your chest and slightly out toward your right elbow.

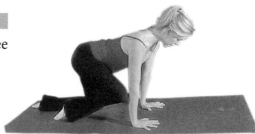

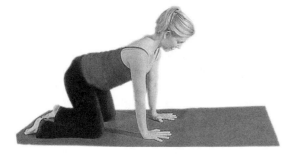

INHALE as you return your knee to the ground. KEEP your neck long and your shoulders wide.

SWITCH legs.

EXHALE as you draw your left leg toward your left elbow. Inhale as you return your left knee to the floor. It is more important to keep your back straight than to bring your knee all the way to your elbow.

This is one set.

Do three sets.

For your review:

Did you need to skip this exercise today?

_____

_____

How did this exercise feel today?

_____

_____

Did you need to modify anything?

_____

_____

Did your baby react more or less today?

_____

_____

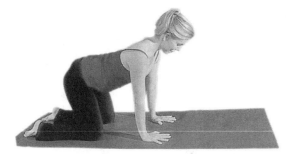

MODIFICATION:

You can kneel on a pillow to give your knees extra cushioning.

TRANSITION:

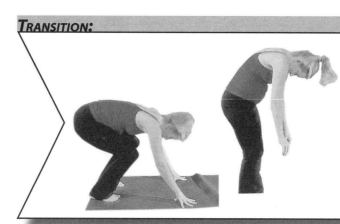

Tuck your toes under. Shift your weight back onto your feet. Roll up, keeping your knees slightly bent. Your head is the last to arrive. Walk over to the wall.

Third Trimester Workout

Leg Circles

What is needed:

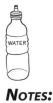

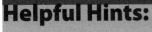

NOTES:

_____

_____

GOAL: To isolate your leg while training the rest of your body to stabilize itself. This stability actually makes the work of the leg easier and lighter.

PRENATAL BENEFITS: Leg strength is important for carrying your body's extra weight comfortably. Being in an upright position allows gravity to work the leg harder. The movement of your leg in the air still helps improve circulation and reduce the swelling that is almost inevitable.

POSITION:

BEGIN standing with your left hand against the wall or the back of a chair for balance. Your right hand is on your hip. Your legs are slightly turned out with your heels together in a **Pilates V.**

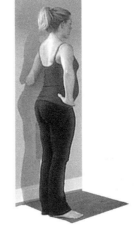

KEEP your **tailbone** reaching down and your **powerhouse** reaching up. This will keep your back long and the weight of your torso out of your legs.

Helpful Hints:

Your hips and torso should remain quiet.

Lift your body off your legs by pulling up from the inside. Imagine children who don't want to be picked up. They let their weight drop to the floor—their little bodies can feel like they weigh 100 pounds! You can control how heavy your body feels to your legs.

The movement comes from the top of your thigh not your foot.

EXECUTION:

INHALE as you raise your straight right leg to a forty-five-degree angle. Without moving any other part of your body, make small circles with the whole leg. Cross the center of your body, then circle down slightly past your body and back to the starting position. Pause at the starting point.

EXHALE for half the circle then inhale for the other half. Try to let your **powerhouse** move your leg.

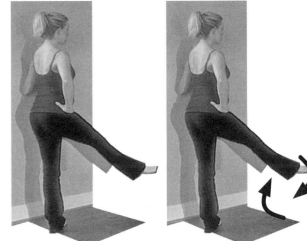

Do five circles, then reverse the direction of the circle five times.

Turn around and repeat the series with your left leg.

For your review:

Did you need to skip this exercise today?

_____

_____

How did this exercise feel today?

_____

_____

Did you need to modify anything?

_____

_____

Did your baby react more or less today?

_____

_____

MODIFICATION:

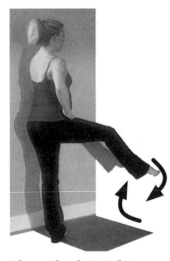

If your back is tight, bend the circling leg.

TRANSITION:

Place your back against the wall.

Stomach Series

What is needed:

WATER

Notes:

_____

_____

_____

_____

The stomach series is designed to target all four abdominal muscle groups. There are five exercises in the series. We will do the first two.

Goal: To work the lower abdominal muscles while stretching your back and legs.

Prenatal Benefits: This is a great way to give your abdominal muscles a little workout without lying on your back. The muscles needed to draw the leg up are the same ones used in delivery. Curling your upper back off the wall while keeping the tailbone reaching down gives your back and leg a much needed stretch.

Single Leg Stretch ⟨4⟩ ⟨5⟩

Position:

STAND with your back against the wall and your feet about six-to-eight inches away from the wall. Your right leg, which you are about to use, will be slightly turned out while your standing left leg is parallel.

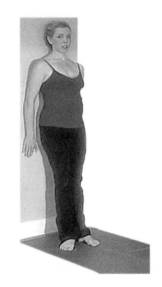

Helpful Hints:

Keep your **tailbone** reaching down to keep your lower back in **neutral**.

Remember to **Kegel** so that the muscles of your **pelvic floor** are used.

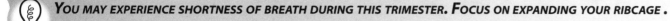

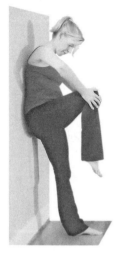

EXECUTION:

EXHALE as you round your upper back forward and raise your right knee. Place your hands on your knee or your thigh. Pulse your leg toward your armpit two times.

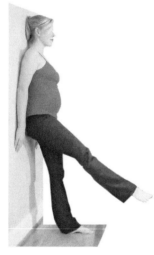

INHALE to lengthen your right leg, still turned out, to a forty-five-degree angle while returning your upper back to the wall. Pull your belly up as your right leg lengthens.

This is one set.

Do four sets. Lower your right leg. Turn it parallel and turn out your left leg.

Do four sets on the left.

MODIFICATION:

If balance is an issue, keep your hands on the wall slightly away from your body. Do not bring them to your knees.

TRANSITION:

Lower your left foot to the floor. Rotate your leg to parallel. Turn out your right foot.

What is needed:

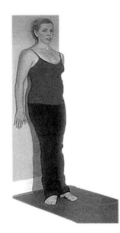

NOTES:

_____

_____

_____

Double Leg Stretch

⚠ 4 ⚠ 5

POSITION:

STAND with your back against the wall and your feet 6-to-8 inches from the wall. Your right leg is turned out while your left leg is parallel. Your arms are at your sides, fingers pointing down.

Helpful Hints:

Don't lock your standing leg.

Draw your belly button and **sternum** into the wall so that your back can round and you can feel more stable.

Don't worry about the height of your leg. Even though your strength and flexibility are improving, your body is continually growing, which will limit your range of motion.

This is the most difficult exercise because of the balance and coordination needed.

If you have trouble with this exercse do a modified version.

Remember to rotate your leg from your hip socket.

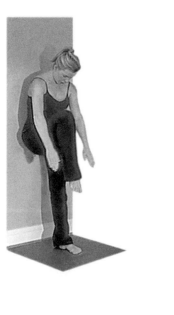

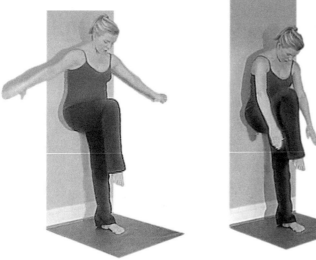

EXECUTION:

EXHALE as you round your upper back off the wall, drawing your knee in the direction of your right armpit as you reach your hands toward your right ankle.

WHILE keeping your upper back curved, inhale and raise your arms over your head. Extend your right leg turned out to a forty-five-degree angle. Take your focus in front of your foot so that your neck will remain long.

EXHALE and circle your arms down as your leg bends in.

This is one set.

Do three sets on the right.

Do three sets on the left.

AT the end of the third set, lower your right leg to the floor. Turn your left leg out and repeat on the other side. Rotate to bend your left leg; inhale to extend it.

MODIFICATION:

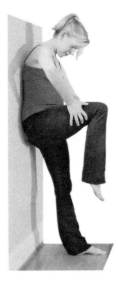

Put your hands on your thigh or knee to assist raising your leg.

For your review:

Did you need to skip this exercise today?

_____

_____

How did this exercise feel today?

_____

_____

Did you need to modify anything?

_____

_____

Did your baby react more or less today?

_____

_____

TRANSITION:

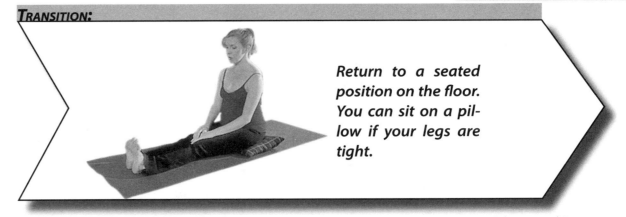

Return to a seated position on the floor. You can sit on a pillow if your legs are tight.

THOUGHTS AND FEELINGS

Date: _____

This time in my pregnancy has been… _____

_____

_____

_____

_____

I feel good about my body because… _____

_____

_____

_____

_____

I am anxious about… _____

_____

_____

_____

Spine Stretch

What is needed:

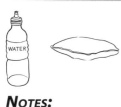

NOTES:

GOAL: To create space between the vertebrae in your spine and teach each vertebra to work independently. This will show you how to find good posture.

PRENATAL BENEFITS: This is a wonderful way to relieve tension in your upper back and shoulders. Remember not to shift forward on your legs. This is not a stretch for the back of the legs (although you may feel a secondary stretch there); it is a spine stretch. Lifting off your hips before moving creates space in the spine, which helps make room for the baby, and allows you space to breathe more comfortably.

POSITION:

SIT on the floor with your legs stretched out in front of you, slightly wider than **hip-width apart.** Raise your arms so they are shoulder-width apart in front of you and parallel to the floor. Feet are relaxed.

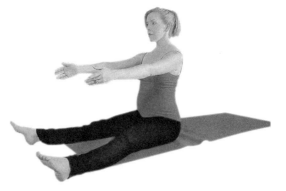

Helpful Hints:

Try sitting against a wall to give you added support and the tactile stimulation needed to tell whether your posture is correct.

Try to get your shoulders, middle back and sacrum to touch the wall.

If you shift too far forward you will get more of a leg stretch. Don't! Remember, this exercise is called **SPINE STRETCH.**

Create as much space between your **vertebrae** so that you make as much room for your baby as possible.

SPINE STRETCH and **CAT** are the best exercises to relieve back and shoulder tension.

EXECUTION:

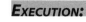

INHALE to grow taller in your spine.

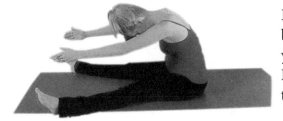

EXHALE. Round forward over your belly, one **vertebra** at a time, beginning with your head. While keeping your head between your arms, reach the crown of your head toward your knees. Keep your shoulders down your back and your arms parallel to the floor.

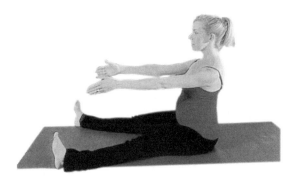

INHALE to begin rolling up.

EXHALE as you finish stacking up your spine; keep your chest open and wide.

This is one set.

Do six sets.

MODIFICATION:

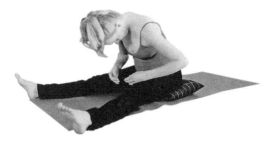

If sitting with your legs straight is uncomfortable, sit on a pillow. You may find you are holding excessive tension in your shoulders with your arms extended. If so, place your arms in your lap but be sure to keep your chest open and your shoulders down.

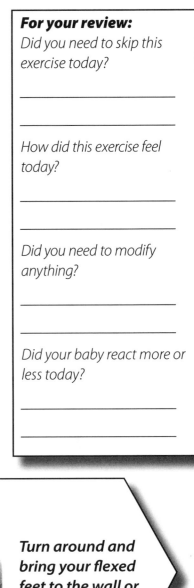

TRANSITION:

Turn around and bring your flexed feet to the wall or couch and close your legs.

MY DELIVERY PLANS

Need to Pack… _Bathrobe, toothpaste, toothbrush, shampoo/conditioner, slippers,_

_____

_____

_____

_____

_____

I hope to deliver at (e.g., home, birthing center, hospital)… _____

_____

_____

_____

_____

My doctor's (midwife's) phone number is… _____

My hospital's, birthing center's phone number is… _____

Twist

What is needed:

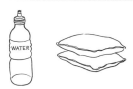

NOTES:

_____

_____

Helpful Hints:

Feel that you are a straight line from elbow to elbow.

Imagine a corkscrew spiraling the cork out of the bottle.

Traditionally the TWIST is done on an exhale. Doing it on an inhale ensures a lift in your torso and limits your risk of over twisting.

Make sure to move smoothly and slowly. No jerky movements.

This is a small and subtle movement. Don't worry about how far you go.

GOAL: To increase spinal rotation and stretch the sides of your torso.

PRENATAL BENEFITS: Your range of motion will be limited now, but this exercise still allows a gentle stretch for your spine and your **obliques.**

POSITION:

SIT with your flexed feet against a wall or stationary object. Your legs are together and long. Your fingertips touch your shoulders; elbows are out, and your chest is open. Your shoulders are drawn down your back. Your back is straight.

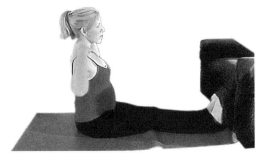

EXECUTION:

MOVING only from your waist up, inhale and lift your **ribcage** off your hips. Twist to the right. Make sure both feet stay on the wall. Twist just from the waist up.

EXHALE to return to center.

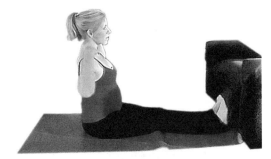

For your review:

Did you need to skip this exercise today?

_____

_____

How did this exercise feel today?

_____

_____

Did you need to modify anything?

_____

_____

Did your baby react more or less today?

_____

_____

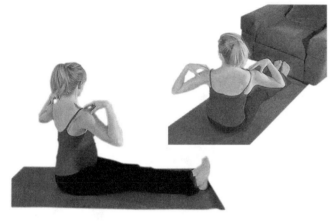

TWIST to the left. Inhale to lift and rotate.

EXHALE to return to center.

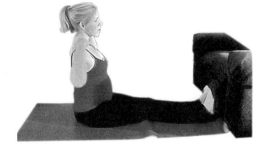

This is one set.

Do three sets.

MODIFICATION:

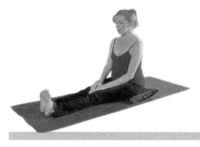

Remain sitting on a pillow if you did so for spine stretch.

Soften your knees but keep your feet flexed and inner thighs glued together.

TRANSITION:

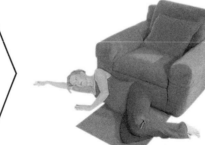

Bend your knees and bring your back to a stationary object. Lie down on your left side.

Side Kick Series

This is a series of leg exercises performed while lying on your side. We will only do two in this series

What is needed:

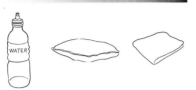

NOTES:

_____

_____

_____

_____

Front/Back

△3 △4 △5

GOAL: To keep your torso completely quiet while moving your legs. This requires abdominal and back strength. You will then be able to stretch your legs and hip flexors gently and correctly.

PRENATAL BENEFITS: This exercise gently worrks your stretched abdominal muscles while lengthening your legs and lower back.

POSITION:

LIE on your left side with your hips and shoulders touching a stationary object. Place a rolled up towel under your head for support. Your left hand is on the floor over your head, palm down, and your right hand is on the floor in front of your s**ternum**.

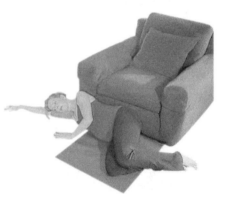

Helpful Hints:

Make sure your leg is slightly higher than hip-width to make room for your belly.

Stick your buttocks out slightly when kicking to the front to keep your **pelvis** from tucking under.

Having a stationary object to back up to will help keep you from kicking too far behind you and over stretching your abdominal wall.

Your torso stays long and connected to the stationary object at all times.

These kicks are done in a controlled and fluid fashion. Do not whack your legs.

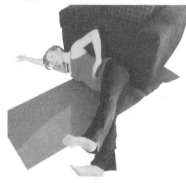

EXTEND your legs in a parallel position out from your hips at a forty-five-degree angle. Both feet are flexed.

INHALE as you lift your left leg slightly higher than hip height.

EXECUTION:

EXHALE as you kick to the front with a double pulse. Keep your torso connected to the stationary object. Make sure your leg is slightly higher than hip-width to make room for your belly.

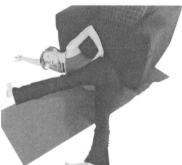

INHALE as you point your foot and kick straight down.

This is one set.

Do eight sets.

MODIFICATION:
Place a pillow or towel under your belly for extra support.

For your review:
Did you need to skip this exercise today?

_____

_____

How did this exercise feel today?

_____

_____

Did you need to modify anything?

_____

_____

Did your baby react more or less today?

_____

_____

TRANSITION:

Remain where you are for the second exercise in the SIDE KICK Series.

Side Kick Series

What is needed:

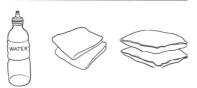

NOTES:

_____

_____

_____

_____

Helpful Hints:

Try not to tuck your pelvis under. Your lower back remains against the stationary object. This will ensure that you are moving within the confines of your body.

Up/Down

⚠3 ⚠4 ⚠5

GOAL: To safely stretch the inner thigh with control and within the limitations of your body.

PRENATAL BENEFITS: Inner thigh strength and flexibility are important if you wish to squat during delivery. Opening the inner thighs and hips helps release and open the pelvic floor enabling the baby to descend more easily through the birth canal.

POSITION:

LYING on your right side, turn your left leg out, point your foot and place your heel on the instep of your right foot.

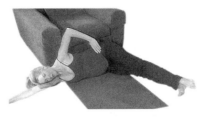

EXECUTION:

EXHALE as you kick your left leg toward the ceiling. Keep your torso long. Make sure you have lots of space for your baby.

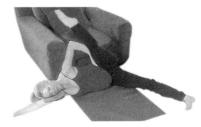

INHALE as you flex your foot and lower your leg back down. Use your inner thigh to control your leg.

This is one set.

Do eight sets.

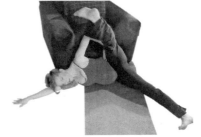
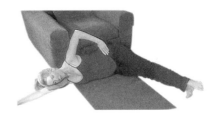

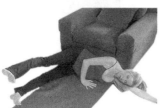

TRANSITION TO LEFT SIDE:

BEND your knees and push up to a seated position. Bring your legs to the other side and slide down the stationary object until you are lying on your left side.

PUT the towel back under your head and place your left hand, palm down, on the floor above your head, and your right hand is on the floor in front of your **sternum.** Make sure that your **sacrum** and shoulders still touch the stationary object.

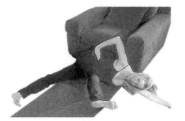

EXECUTION ON LEFT SIDE:

Using your right leg do eight sets of FRONT/BACK

and

UP/DOWN.

MODIFICATION:

Place a pillow or rolled up towel under your belly for added support. Even then, make sure you are using your own muscles to support your belly.

For your review:

Did you need to skip this exercise today?

_____

_____

How did this exercise feel today?

_____

_____

Did you need to modify anything?

_____

_____

Did your baby react more or less today?

_____

_____

TRANSITION:

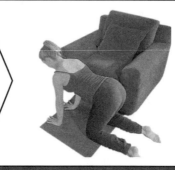

Bend both legs and push up to a seated position. Come onto your hands and knees with one side of your body touching the stationary object or wall.

Swimming

What is needed:

WATER

NOTES:

_____

_____

_____

_____

GOAL: To strengthen the muscles in your back.

PRENATAL BENEFIT: Your back will need to be extra strong to counterbalance your growing belly. Poor posture leads to back pain, as I'm sure you have already discovered!

POSITION:

You are in a hands and knees position with your hands directly under your shoulders and your knees under your hips. Your back is long and straight with your belly well supported.

EXECUTION:

INHALE to reach your right arm long to float up parallel to the floor. Make sure your shoulder stays drawn down your back.

EXHALE as you lower your arm back down to it's starting position. Try to touch the floor as far away from you as you can without allowing your shoulder to come forward.

KEEP your neck and torso long.

Helpful Hints:

Press into your palms and pull them back slightly without moving your hands. This will help keep shoulders wide and drawn down your back.

Imagine your abdominal muscles are cradling your baby so that you do not sink into your lower back.

As much as your arm and leg reach away from one another, your shoulder and hip draw toward each other. This oppositional pull will give you power and aid in balance.

Having one side of your body against something stationary will help your balance. Try alternating which side you place against the wall each time you do this exercise.

PRACTICE TENSING, THEN COMPLETELY RELEASING YOUR MUSCLES AS A WAY TO RELIEVE TENSION.

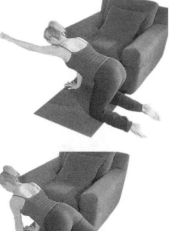

REPEAT using your left arm. Let your back initiate this motion.

INHALE as you slide your right foot until it floats off the floor. Make sure your belly is supported.

EXHALE as you reach your leg back down to the floor and bend it back in.

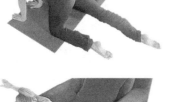

REPEAT using your left leg. Try not to shift in your hips. Your hip will want to sink as your leg moves. Use your back muscles to keep your torso on one plane.

INHALE as you reach your right arm and left leg away from your torso until they float off the floor.

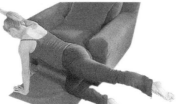

EXHALE and lower your arm and leg at the same time.

REPEAT using your left arm and right leg.

Do two sets of your arm and leg reaching up together.

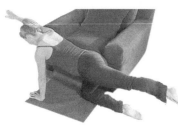

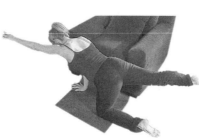

TRANSITION:

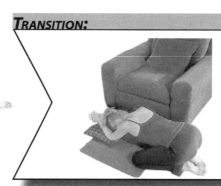

Shift your weight back onto your heels while opening your knees wide enough to accommodate your baby. Rest your arms and head on a pillow for added support.

Child's Pose/A Little Piece of Heaven

What is needed:

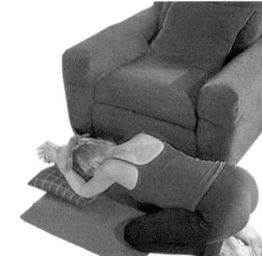

NOTES:

_____

_____

_____

_____

_____

GOAL: To release the muscles in your back.

PRENATAL BENEFITS: Pregnant women are prone to lower backaches. This pose doesn't require any warm up and you can practice the very important **PILATES BREATHING** technique in a position that will allow your breath to open up your back.

POSITION:

SIT back on your heels with your feet together and your knees wider than **hip width** to make room for your belly. Rest your head and your arms on a pillow.

EXECUTION:

THE hardest things you have to do here are relax and practice your **BREATHING**. Imagine breathing into your back. Feel your lower and mid back open up and release.

Helpful Hints:

Do this pose whenever you feel strain or tension in your lower back.

For your review:

Did you need to skip this exercise today?

_____

_____

How did this exercise feel today?

_____

_____

Did you need to modify anything?

_____

_____

Did your baby react more or less today?

_____

_____

CHILD'S POSE is an exercise taken from yoga. **Pilates** aptly renamed it, **"A LITTLE PIECE OF HEAVEN"** because that is what it feels like!

STAY through six deep breaths. If you wish, you can always return to this position at the end of your workout.

MODIFICATION:

If you have knee problems, place a pillow behind your knees before shifting back to take the strain off your knees.

TRANSITION:

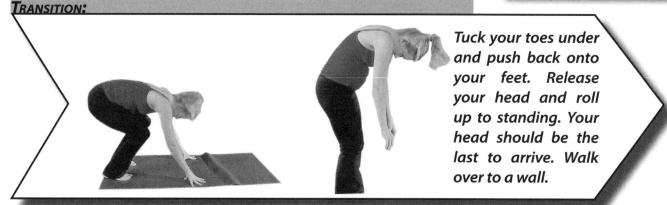

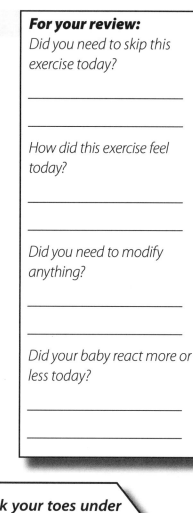

Tuck your toes under and push back onto your feet. Release your head and roll up to standing. Your head should be the last to arrive. Walk over to a wall.

Flat Back Punches

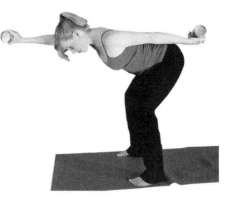

What is needed:

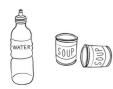

NOTES:

_____

_____

_____

_____

GOAL: To strengthen your back.

PRENATAL BENEFITS: A stronger back improves your posture.

POSITION:

STAND with your feet slightly wider than **hip-width apart** while holding one soup can in each hand. Bend forward from your waist until your torso is parallel to the floor. Soften your knees. Keep your back flat and your focus to the floor. Bring your torso up if your back rounds. Bend your arms and keep them tight against your body.

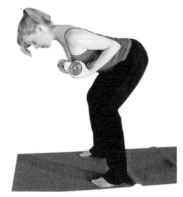

EXECUTION:

INHALE as you punch your right arm to the front, palm down and your left arm to the back, palm up. Make sure your arms stay in line with your torso.

Helpful Hints:

Support your belly and stick your tailbone out to keep your back flat.

Reach your arms long in opposition while keeping your shoulders down.

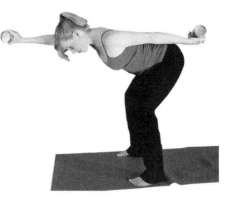

READ A GOOD BOOK – WHILE YOU STILL HAVE EXTRA TIME!

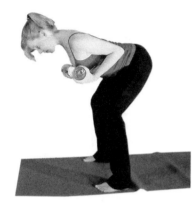

EXHALE as you bend your arms back.

SWITCH arms:

PUNCH your left arm to the front and your right to the back.

This is one set.

Do four sets.

For your review:

Did you need to skip this exercise today?

_____

_____

How did this exercise feel today?

_____

_____

Did you need to modify anything?

_____

_____

Did your baby react more or less today?

_____

_____

TRANSITION:

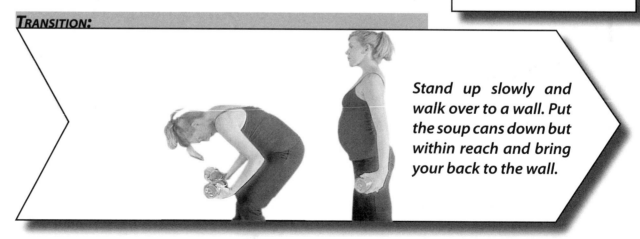

Stand up slowly and walk over to a wall. Put the soup cans down but within reach and bring your back to the wall.

Round Down with Push Up

What is needed:

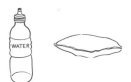

NOTES:

_____

_____

_____

_____

GOAL: To stretch your back and strengthen your arms.

PRENATAL BENEFITS: Doing **tricep** pushups in this modified position allows you to get a great upper body and arm workout without undue strain on your back and belly. Rolling down and up against the wall allows you to feel each vertebra to make sure to make sure that your lower spine is not overly arched. **ROUND DOWN** allows you to get a great stretch in the muscles of your back and legs.

POSITION:

STAND with your back against a wall with your feet parallel, about six inches from the wall and wider than **hip-width apart**. There may be a very small space behind your lower back, but everything else should be touching.

EXECUTION:

INHALE as you bring your arms over your head. Make sure to keep your back in contact with the wall.

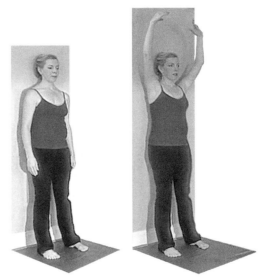

Helpful Hints:

Lift up and draw your spine into the wall before peeling it off. You may need to soften your knees in order to get your lower back to melt into the wall. Your head is the first to leave the wall and the last to return.

Imprint your spine into the wall as you roll down and up.

There is more of an up and over feeling than just a forward motion.

Keep your neck and shoulders relaxed as you roll down or up.

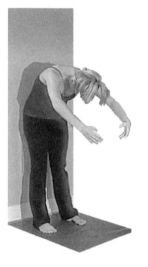

EXHALE as you peel each **vertebra** off the wall, one at a time, and roll all the way down.

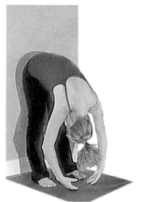

INHALE at the bottom and walk your hands out as you lower your knees to the floor.

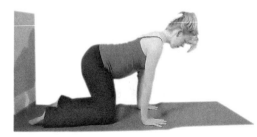

COME to a hands and knees position.

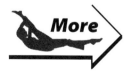
More

KEEPING your arms tight to your body, exhale as you bend your arms. Your head will lower to the floor with your back on a diagonal.

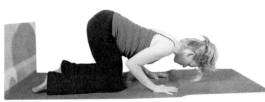

Do not shift back. Your chest should stay over your hands. Make sure your belly is supported and you do not sink into your lower back and shoulders.

INHALE as you straighten your arms.

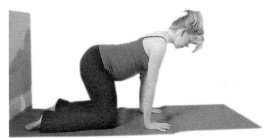

This is one push up.

Do three of these modified push ups.

EXHALE to shift back and tuck your toes under. Inhale and push back onto your feet.

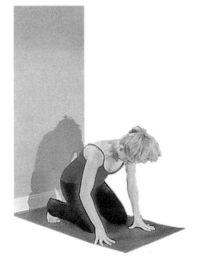

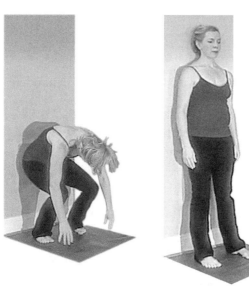

EXHALE to roll all the way back to standing, getting each **vertebra** on the wall, one at a time. Your head is the last to arrive.

This is one set.

Do three sets with three push ups each.

MODIFICATION:

Place a pillow under your knees for the push up.

If this push up is too difficult today, just bend your arms slightly. Or skip the push up all together. Simply roll down and up against the wall.

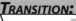
TRANSITION:

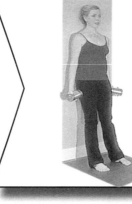

Pick up two soup cans and return your back to the wall. Walk your feet even further away so that when you bend your knees they do not go past your feet.

Curls

What is needed:

NOTES:

_____

_____

_____

GOAL: To strengthen the arms, legs and buttocks.

PRENATAL BENEFITS: This exercise builds stamina, which you may need during labor. It also strengthens your legs so that they can carry your greater weight more easily. The arm strength developed here is vital for the not too distant future when you have a baby to carry all day long.

POSITION:

STAND against a wall with your legs parallel and your feet slightly wider than **hip-width apart,** holding a soup can (or one- to-three pound weight) with each hand. Your feet are far enough from the wall so that your knees will be directly over your feet when you bend your knees and come into a seated position. Inhale to lower your body into an "invisible chair". You may need to readjust your feet to ensure proper alignment.

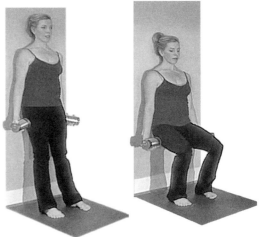

Helpful Hints:

Make sure you are barefoot or standing on a nonslip surface.

Imprint your spine into the wall.

Stay lifted in your torso without lifting your shoulders. The more you can support your body by lifting through your torso, the less strain you will feel in your legs.

This exercise will get harder as you get bigger. You may need to adjust how deeply you sit.

EXECUTION:

Do four **BICEP CURLS.**

EXHALE as you bend your arms. Inhale as your arms lengthen. Keep your focus directly in front of you. The back of your neck remains long. Finish on an exhale.

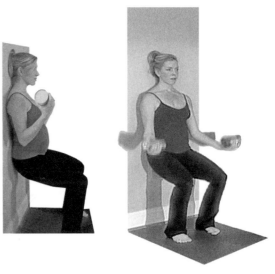

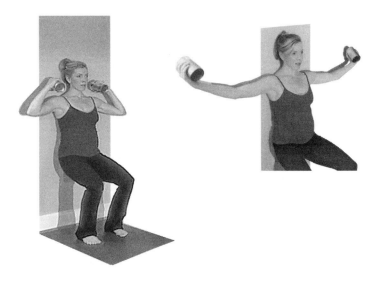

EXHALE to raise your elbows to the side, shoulder height, arms bent and against the wall. Do four more **bicep** curls with your arms against the wall.

INHALE as you lengthen your arms.

FINISH on an exhale.

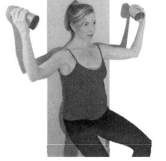 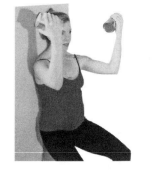

INHALE to open your arms to a ninety-degree angle.

Do four repetions closing and opening your arms in front of you.

EXHALE as you close your arms in front of your chest. Inhale to open your arms to the wall.

FINISH on an inhale.

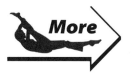

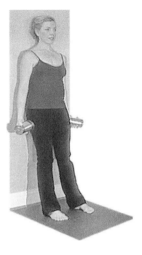

EXHALE to straighten your legs and lower your arms.

TAKE a brief break.

This is one full set of CURLS.

Do two sets of all three CURLS.

MODIFICATION:

Only bend your knees slightly if you have knee problems or you feel weak in your legs.

You can choose to keep your legs straight and only do the CURLS or bend your legs without the weights and work on your **breathing technique**.

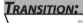

TRANSITION:

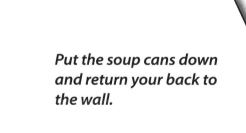

Put the soup cans down and return your back to the wall.

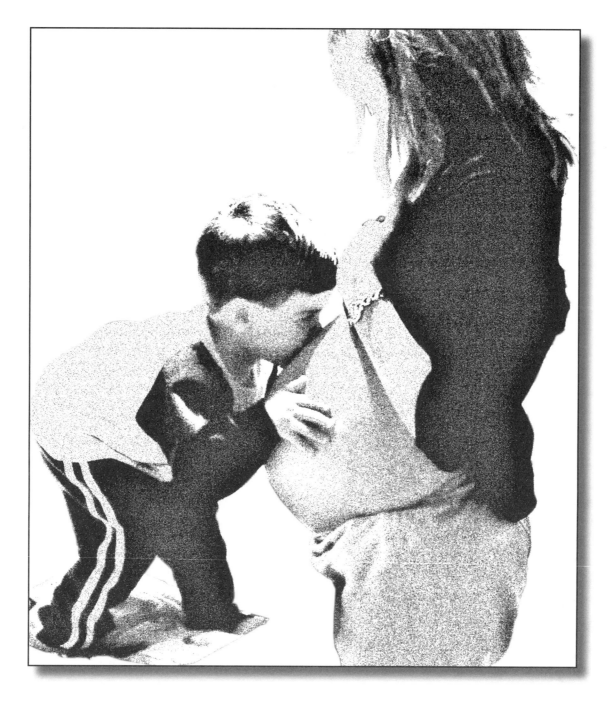

Squat

What is needed:

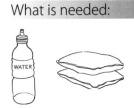

NOTES:

_____

_____

_____

_____

GOAL: To stretch your calves and inner thighs while opening up your pelvis.

PRENATAL BENEFITS: This position opens the pelvic floor and facilitates the descent and passage of your baby through the birth canal.

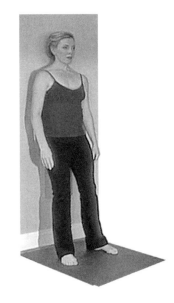

POSITION:

YOUR back is securely against a wall and your feet about six-to-eight inches away. Your legs are wider than **hip-width apart.** Your legs and feet are slightly turned out.

Helpful Hints:

Remember to take the last few weeks off to rest. Choose a few of the relaxation poses like CHILD'S POSE, SPINE STRETCH and ROUND DOWN without push up, to get you through the last few weeks.

EXECUTION:

IMPRINT your back against the wall. Inhale then exhale and slide as far down as you can, using the wall for support. Your heels remain on the ground.

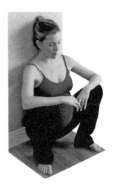

Pilates and Pregnancy

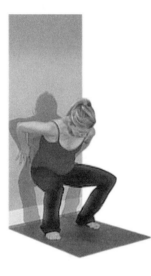

FEEL your inner thighs open up. Just breathe. Relax into this stretch.

REMEMBER to inhale through your nose, exhale out your mouth.

AFTER six breaths, walk your hands up the wall to help you stand.

COME away from the wall. Stand with your heels together, toes slightly apart in a **Pilates V.** Support your belly and feel your lower back lengthen. Shoulders are relaxed and your neck is long. Try to remember this feeling for the rest of the day.

MODIFICATION:

If this position is uncomfortable, try sitting on one or two pillows.

For your review:

Did you need to skip this exercise today?

_____

_____

How did this exercise feel today?

_____

_____

Did you need to modify anything?

_____

_____

Did your baby react more or less today?

_____

_____

WEIGHT AT THE BEGINNING OF THE 3RD TRIMESTER: _____

WEIGHT AT THE END OF THE 3RD TRIMESTER: _____

BLOOD PRESSURE AT THE BEGINNING OF THE 3RD TRIMESTER: _____

BLOOD PRESSURE AT THE END OF THE 3RD TRIMESTER: _____

TEST/RESULTS: _____

HOW DOES YOUR BODY FEEL? _____ *BACK PAIN?* _____ *SCIATICA?* _____ *TIGHTNESS?* _____

DID ANY EXERCISES FEEL ESPECIALLY GOOD? _____ *HOW?* _____

DID YOU AVOID OR MODIFY ANY EXERCISES? _____ *WHY?* _____

HOW MANY DAYS PER WEEK DID YOU DO PILATES AND PREGNANCY? _____

HOW MANY DAYS PER WEEK DID YOU DO LIGHT CARDIO? _____

DATE: _____

Section II: Machine Exercises

Notes for Machine Work

Please note that all machine work should be done under the supervision and guidance of a certified Pilates instructor. The suggested machine exercises in this section and the various modifications are written for your instructor. A trained eye, experienced spotting and assistance during some exercises make working out with a qualified teacher essential when doing machine work while pregnant. Since your sense of balance will change as your pregnancy progresses, spotting is required for standing and some kneeling exercises. I have noted which exercises need your teacher to keep her hands on you.

Anytime you feel strain or pulling in the abdominal region, stop. Note the modifications for the springs. Sometimes you will need lighter springs; sometimes you will need more assistance. You can move the gear bar back or open your legs wider to give yourself more space when seated.

Always keep you belly well supported by not sinking into your back. Your instructor may wish to keep her/his hand on your belly as a reminder and for added support.

Realize that your range of motion (ROM) will be limited to prevent overstretching your abdominal muscles and ligaments. Even your wrists may be more sensitive. Take a break in between exercises that are weight bearing on your hands. The hormone Relaxin will make your joints much looser so take it slow!

I have given modifications for second and third trimesters on the Cadillac, Low Chair and Reformer. The modifications from the second trimester exercises carry over to the third trimester. During your first trimester, do what is comfortable. However, now is not the time to try something new and difficult.

It may be challenging to find a teacher who has had prenatal Pilates training. If you do find someone willing to work with you during your pregancy, I recommend taking this book with you to your session. And make sure your instructor is certified on the Pilates equipment.

All workouts should be one on one. I do not recommend group classes.

Focus on your breath throughout your workout. The more you can expand your ribcage during your inhalations the easier it will be to take full and deep breathes later in your pregnancy. Pilates can help you feel relaxed, reduce swelling in your legs and feet and alleviate back pain. You should sleep well tonight!

Machine Exercises For Pregnancy

REFORMER EXERCISES	2ND TRIMESTER	3RD TRIMESTER
Rowing 1-6	rowing 3-6 / light spring	shave and hug a tree/light spring
Horseback	light spring/ spot for balance	no springs or straps/fists on box behind you
Elephant	spot for balance	knees soft/ spot
Long back stretch	if wrists are ok	if wrists are ok
stomach massage	1 less spring	gear bar back/feet apart
Tendon Stretch	legs apart/ assist coming in	all springs/just stretch and sit/spot
chest expansion	light spring/spot	sitting on box face back
thigh stretch	small ROM	spot and assist coming up
The Hundred	sitting/pumping rolldown bar in front	use light lighter bar or magic circle
mermaid	1 leg in front	move gear back/ small ROM
short box	Side Bend/ Twist on inhale/ beginning of tree	Side Bend/ small Twist on inhale
knee stretches	no knees off	move gear bar back
side splits	spot	spot
gondola	spot	spot
eves lunge	move gear	move gear

CADILLAC EXERCISES	2ND TRIMESTER	3RD TRIMESTER
Roll down	knees bent	knees bent/help up
Cat	normal	1/2 way but still extend

CADILLAC EXERCISES (CONTINUED)	2ND TRIMESTER	3RD TRIMESTER
thigh stretch	spot and assist coming up	spot and assist coming up
push through	push the bar	legs turned out
shoulder abduction/ adduction	standing with arm spring	with arm spring
side leg springs	limit ROM	pillow under stomach

CHAIR EXERCISES	2ND TRIMESTER	3RD TRIMESTER
footwork	smaller ROM	hip-width/ 2nd position
Pumping	smaller ROM	2nd position
foot and ankle exercise	normal	pillow under knee if necessary
standing pumping	standing knee bent	lighter spring/spot
spine stretch	light spring	light spring
low frog	incline	no chair/ heels together/ round over
standing push down	hip width	wider
standing push down behind	small box under pedal/hold hips	no
cat	box under pedal/ hold feet	wider knees
mermaid/ side arm sit	small ROM	Just touch pedal
arm press plie	light spring	support under arms
triceps press	small ROM	small ROM
Lunges	heavy spring/hold handles	wider base

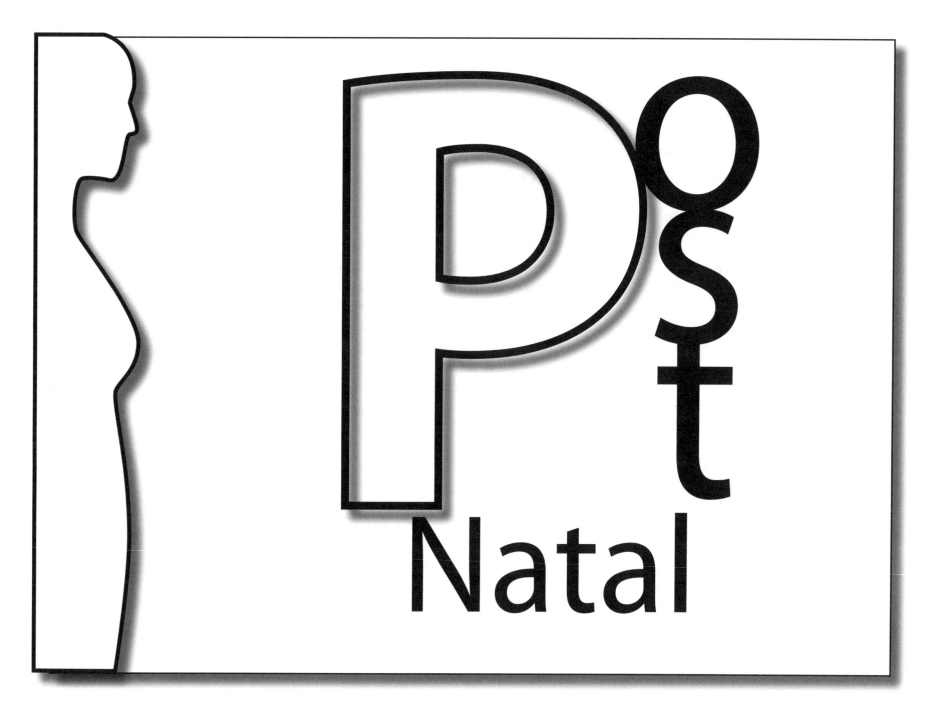

Post
Natal

Referring to Sarah Picot's Post-natal Pilates DVD containing the companion exercises to this book, Dr. Collin Cullen writes:

"I have just finished viewing POST-NATAL PILATES. After watching the video, it is abundant in the facial interaction and soothing touch that are so necessary for early mother and child bonding: this is combined with an exercise program geared towards the new mother, whose temporal and emotional constraints are an important issue. I think that children in this perinatal period are very responsive to tactile, auditory and visual stimuli and with the mother's ability to interact with the child during this work-out makes this a far superior exercise tape in the postnatal period as compared to those that do not try to incorporate these concerns. After viewing the tape, I could confidently and enthusiastically recommend it to my new, and experienced, mothers to use to maximize their small and valuable time to get the exercise the body needs and continue to encourage and foster the bonding relationship that mother (and father) and baby need."

Sincerely,

Collin D. Cullen, M.D.
Board Certified Internal Medicine
Board Certified Pediatrics

Post-Natal Workout

Congratulations! All of your hard work and discipline paid off. You now have the reward in your arms.

You may be feeling sore, tired or even experiencing some mild post-partum depression. It's all very normal. Thankfully these symptoms lessen with time. Besides the benefits to your body, exercise also helps your emotions; it makes you feel better. The increased oxygen and blood flow along with any endorphins (a chemical released during exercise and excitement) can help you mentally as well as physically. But if you experience more than mild depression or if it lasts for more than a week, consult your doctor.

The aches and pains will go away, but how will you find time to work out with a baby who needs constant attention and supervision? Make your baby part of the workout!

The exercises in this book have been modified to incorporate your baby. When your baby is younger, he can lie on your chest and stomach (a) and hear the soothing sound of your heartbeat. This is comforting because it is the same sound he listened to while in utero. When he is older and more comfortable in a seated position, you can support your baby as she sits on your stomach. This will help remind you to keep your abdominal muscles pulled in and allow her a different view of the room while enjoying your touch. Some of the exercises allow your baby to lean back on your legs (b). This added weight increases the difficulty of the exercise while giving your baby the opportunity to stay close to you.

For many of the exercises your baby will be lying in a supportive pillow or bouncy seat next to you. Your baby will love watching you, while she follows the move-

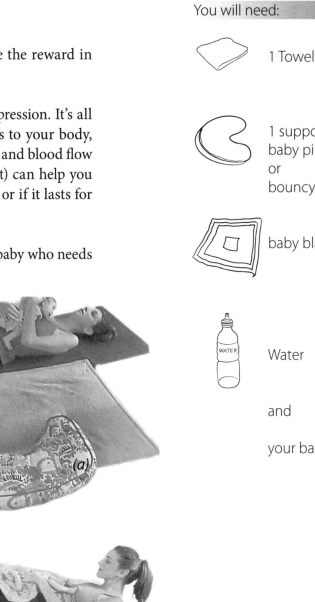

(a)

(b)

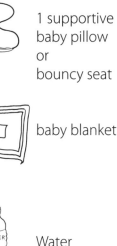

1 Towel

1 supportive
baby pillow
or
bouncy seat

baby blanket

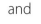

Water

and

your baby!

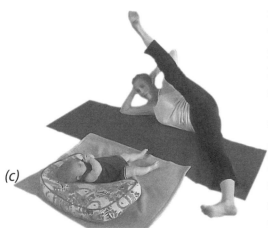

ment of your body. This skill is called tracking (c). When babies are very young they assume that when an object is out of their sight, it has disappeared. When you leave her vision briefly and then reappear she is learning about object permanence (d). You can turn it into a game of peek-a-boo. Don't worry that your baby is just lying next to you. She is getting plenty of visual, mental and emotional stimulation.

(c)

Only you know your baby. If music is soothing or a favorite toy makes her smile, use it. If she doesn't like lying on her back put her stomach. If she gets fussy during a particular exercise, skip it or try placing her in the supportive pillow next to you with a favorite toy. Make this fun! Tickles, making faces and talking to your baby will make exercising more enjoyable for you as well as your baby. Remember, the object is to keep your baby close and entertained so that you can work out while bonding with your baby.

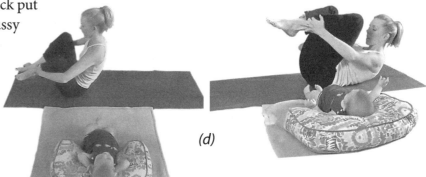

(d)

This program is geared for a two-to-six month old baby. After about six months, your baby will be too active and weigh too much. Note that

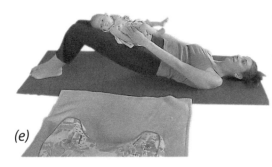

(e)

the age of your baby, along with your baby's preferences will dictate her position on you. A newborn baby will lie back on your legs or on your stomach (e) but not sit up. An older baby who can lift and support his head, may be more comfortable in an upright position with you securely supporting his back and neck (f). When your baby is older than six months or crawling these exercises can be done more traditionally without your baby as long as he is safely in a playpen in the room with you.

You may need to stop to feed or soothe your baby. You may also need to stop to drink some water or go to the bathroom. Remember, water is crucial for healing and breast milk production. So keep plenty of water within reach. However, try not to stop abruptly. Quick, jarring movement isn't good for you or your baby.

If tender breasts make stomach lying uncomfortable, try planning your workouts a half hour after a feeding when your breasts are less full.

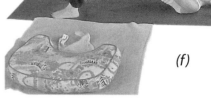

(f)

Safety comes first. Anytime your baby is lying or sitting on you, you must have at least one hand securely holding him. If he is too wriggly today, place him in a bouncy seat or lay him on the supportive pillow next to you. But be sure he is out of reach of your arms and legs.

Before you begin this or any other exercise program, get permission from your doctor. Most women can begin doing abdominal exercise six weeks postpartum, whether you delivered vaginally or via cesarean section. But every woman is different. A c-section may require you to place your baby next to you rather than on your stomach until the incision site feels less tender.

Please note that a **diastasis** (separation) of the **rectus abdominus** muscle of two fingers or more will require you to work out as if you were still in your third trimester to prevent making the condition worse. You can keep your baby at your side but continue with the third trimester workout. Focus on the **obliques** and **tranverses** until your condition is corrected.

Keep some toys, a bouncy chair or supportive pillow and a soft blanket ready for your baby. You will need to dress in comfortable clothes and have your water at the ready.

Now go have some fun with your baby!

Bridging

▲1 ▲2 ▲3 ▲4 ▲5

What is needed:

WATER

NOTES:

_____

_____

_____

_____

Helpful Hints:

Pull your inner thighs toward each other to keep your legs from rolling out.

Try to keep your buttocks lifted as you melt your **sternum** and mid back into the floor.

GOAL: To massage your back and stretch your quadriceps and hip flexors.

POST-NATAL BENEFIT: This exercise helps return your lower back to better alignment. Your baby will love going for a ride.

POSITION:

LIE on your back with your legs bent, **hip-width apart,** and your feet flat on the floor. Sit your baby on your **pelvis** and hold him securely with both hands.

✱KEEP a supportive pillow or bouncy seat close by in case you choose to do an exercise without your baby.

EXECUTION:

INHALE as you tilt your **pubic bone** toward the ceiling, and melt your back into the floor.

EXHALE as you continue to roll up one **vertebra** at a time, all the while drawing your belly button toward your spine.

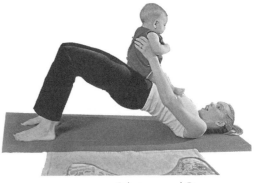

Pilates and Pregnancy

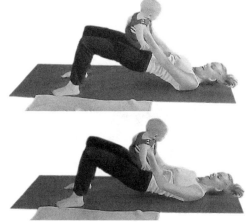

INHALE at the top.

EXHALE and roll all the way down one vertebra at a time.

This is is one set.

Do four sets.

MODIFICATION:

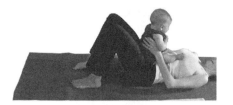

If your baby is younger or not stable in a seated position, close your legs and lean her back against your thighs. You may not be able to come up as high with your legs together. This modification makes your inner thighs work harder and stretches your **quadriceps** and **hip flexors** more intensely.

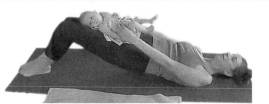

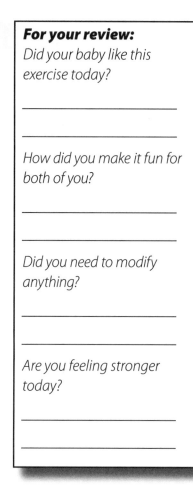

For your review:

Did your baby like this exercise today?

_____

_____

How did you make it fun for both of you?

_____

_____

Did you need to modify anything?

_____

_____

Are you feeling stronger today?

_____

_____

TRANSITION:

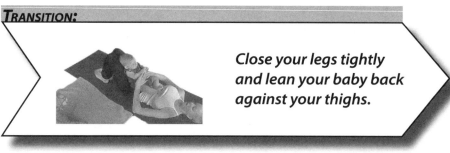

Close your legs tightly and lean your baby back against your thighs.

The Hundred

What is needed:

NOTES:

_____

_____

_____

_____

GOAL: To increase overall circulation and to strengthen your **powerhouse.**

POST-NATAL BENEFITS: Increased oxygen and blood flow will help speed up the healing process. Your baby will enjoy looking at your face and being close to you..

POSITION:

LIE on your back, knees bent, feet flat on the floor and your legs closed tightly together. Your baby is leaning back on your thighs, with your left hand holding her securely. Your right arm is extended long at your side and off the floor a few inches.

CURL your head and shoulders off the ground and extend your right leg. Your right leg is turned out with both knees and inner thighs glued together.

Helpful Hints:

Pump your arms from your back. The rhythm of your arms should dictate the tempo of your breath.

Keep your belly pulled in and up.

The weight of your baby against your thighs will make this exercise even harder than the traditional HUNDREDS. Even if you feel strong, start with the easiest modification of feet and upper back down, then raise your head and shoulders, then lift one leg. Only when you are really strong and do not let your abdominal muscles push out, should you lift both legs.

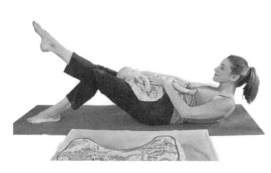

EXECUTION:

WHILE pumping your straight arm up and down, inhale through your nose for five counts, exhale out your mouth for five counts.

This is one set.

Do five sets, then switch sides:

MAINTAIN your position as you place your right hand on your baby. Parallel and bend your right leg in.

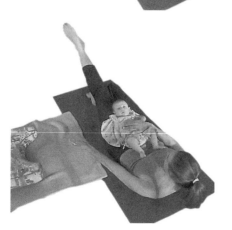

EXTEND your left leg turned out while extending your left arm.

Do five sets using your left arm and leg.

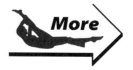

More

MODIFICATIONS:

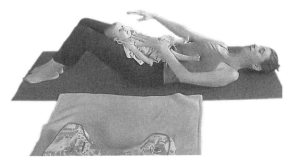

Keep both feet on the floor with your legs together. You may even keep your head and shoulders down if you feel tense. Work on your **BREATHING TECHNIQUE**.

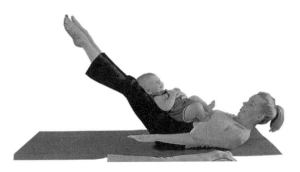

ADVANCED: If you are a level 5 and feel very strong, you can extend both legs turned out slightly past ninety-degrees. Continue to hold the baby with one hand. Switch hands when you transition from the first five sets to the second.

For your review:

Did your baby like this exercise today?

_____

_____

How did you make it fun for both of you?

_____

_____

Did you need to modify anything?

_____

_____

Are you feeling stronger today?

_____

_____

TRANSITION:

Place both hands on your baby. Lower your feet to the floor. Flex your feet.

THOUGHTS AND FEELINGS

Date: _____

This time with my baby has been... _____

_____

_____

_____

_____

I feel good about my body because... _____

_____

_____

_____

_____

I am anxious about... _____

_____

_____

_____

Roll Up

What is needed:

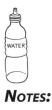

NOTES:

_____

_____

Helpful Hints:

Go through a **pelvic tilt** as you roll up and down to get your lower back on the floor.

Your baby will help remind you with little kicks to keep your belly pulled in and your back round.

Let your baby's legs extend up your stomach as you ROLL UP.

Smile and enjoy the face to face contact at the top of ROLL UP. Take a moment to tickle her as you lower your arm to your thigh.

GOAL: To tone your **powerhouse** while stretching your back.

POST-NATAL BENEFITS: This exercise targets and flattens your stomach. Your baby will enjoy a gentle rocking motion.

POSITION:

LIE on your back with your legs bent and pressed tightly together, feet flexed. Your left hand is behind your left thigh.

YOUR baby is leaning back against your thighs with your right hand holding him securely.

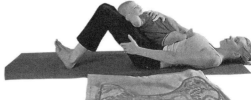

EXECUTION:

INHALE to curl your head and shoulders off the floor.

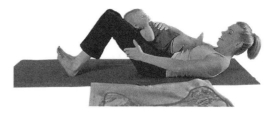

EXHALE and continue to roll up, one **vertebra** at a time.

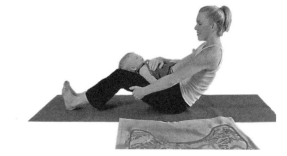

EXTEND your legs long and reach your left arm out, parallel to the floor. You will be sitting with your back in C curve, belly scooped in. Make room for your baby.

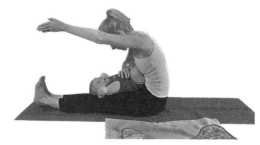

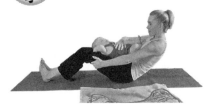

INHALE as you prepare to roll down, lowering your left hand to your thigh.

EXHALE and draw your belly away from your thighs and pull your back into the ground, bending your knees as you go.

UNCURL all the way down.

This is one set.

Do three sets.

SWITCH sides:

PLACE your left hand on your baby before putting your right hand behind your right thigh.

Do three more sets while holding your right thigh.

✳Make sure your left hand stays on your baby.

MODIFICATION:

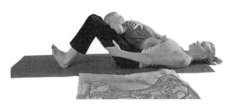

Only come part way up, but focus on curling your spine and keeping your belly pulled in and up.

If your baby doesn't like this today or he is wriggling too much, place him in the supportive pillow next to you and place both hands behind your thighs.

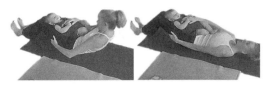

For your review:

Did your baby like this exercise today?

_____

_____

How did you make it fun for both of you?

_____

_____

Did you need to modify anything?

_____

_____

Are you feeling stronger today?

_____

_____

TRANSITION:

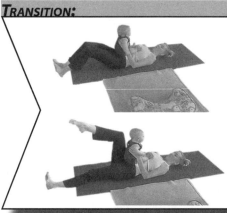

Place both hands on your baby and sit her upright on your lower abdomen and pelvis. Extend your left leg all the way only the floor. Foot flexed. Float your right leg to chair position.

Leg Circles

What is needed:

WATER

NOTES:

_____

_____

_____

Helpful Hints:

Keep your belly button reaching for your spine.

Relax your working foot so that your **quadriceps** will be less likely to engage.

Keep the circles small and within the confines of your body.

The weight of your baby will help remind you to keep your **pelvis** quiet and your hips even.

GOAL: To learn to move your leg independently from the rest of your body.

POST-NATAL BENEFITS: LEG CIRCLES help strengthen the pelvic girdle that has shifted and loosened in order for you to deliver your baby. Your baby will enjoy looking at your face.

POSITION:

LIE on your back with your left leg straight along the floor, foot flexed. Extend your right leg, turned out, toward the ceiling, foot relaxed.

BOTH of your hands are on your baby since he is seated on your lower abdomen. Your elbows can bend so that your upper arms are on the floor.

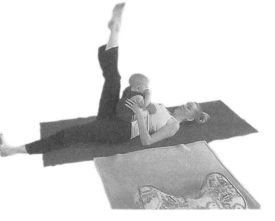

EXECUTION:

WITHOUT moving your torso, make *small* circles with your whole leg. Circle your right leg across your body, slightly down, around and up to the starting position. Inhale as you begin your circle, exhale as you complete it. Pause at the starting position each time.

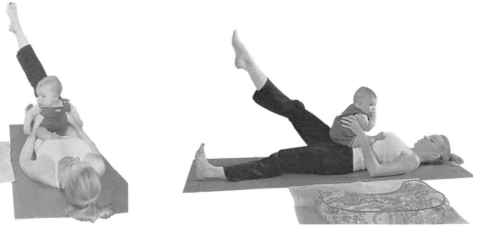
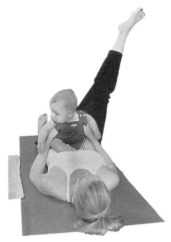

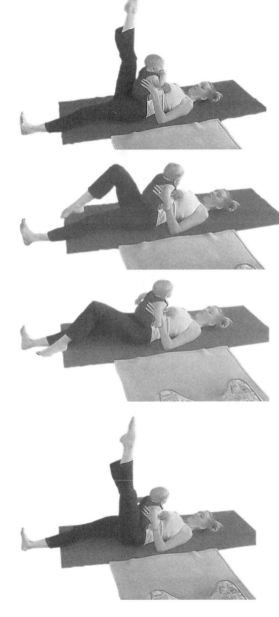

Make five circles in one direction, then reverse the direction of the circle for five.

CHANGE legs.

BEND your right leg and place your right foot on the floor. Extend your right leg along the floor and flex your right foot.

BEND your left leg to **chair position** and extend your left leg to the ceiling, foot relaxed.

Do five circles in each direction using your left leg.

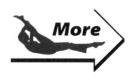
More

MODIFICATION:

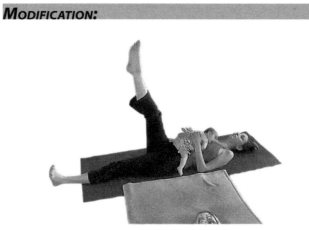

If your baby isn't ready to sit up, lay her on your stomach.

TRANSITION:

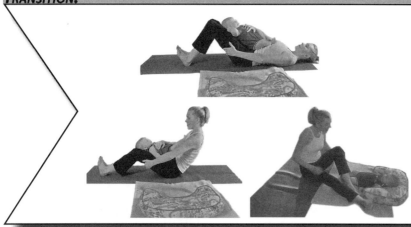

Turn your left leg parallel, bend it and lower your foot to the ground. Point your right foot and bend your leg back in. Close your legs tightly.

Rest your baby against your thighs. Place your right hand on your baby and your left hand behind your thigh.

Do one good ROLL UP.

Place your baby on the supportive pillow or bouncy seat next to you.

Leave some space between the two of you.

A Letter to My Baby

Date: _____

Dear Baby… _____

_____

_____

_____

_____

_____

_____

_____

_____

_____

_____

_____

_____

_____

_____

Rolling Like a Ball

What is needed:

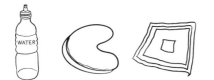

NOTES:

_____

_____

_____

_____

GOAL: To massage your spine.

POST-NATAL BENEFITS: This exercise helps round your lower back and relieve backache. Your baby gets to play a game of peek-a-boo while learning about object permanence—when an object leaves your sight it hasn't disappeared.

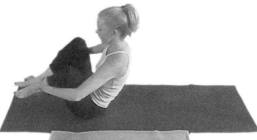

POSITION:

SIT in a curved-back position or capital C, with your pelvis tucked under. Your heels are together, knees in line with your shoulders. Your hands are on your shins.

YOUR baby is on a supportive pillow at your side.

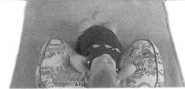

Helpful Hints:

Keep your feet off the floor throughout the exercise.

Try to keep your feet close to your buttocks.

Focus just in front of your feet.

Pretend that you are still nine months pregnant and need to make room for your belly by pulling away from your thighs.

Your roll should be smooth.

Take a moment while you are balanced to look at and talk to your baby.

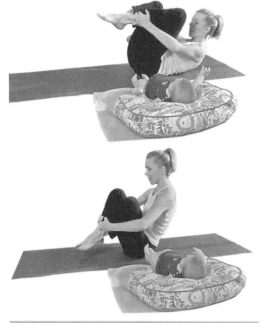

EXECUTION:

WITHOUT rolling onto your neck and shoulders, roll back and up. Inhale to go back. Exhale to roll up. Balance at the top.

This is one set.

Do five sets.

MODIFICATION:

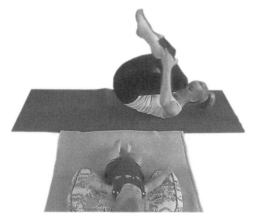

Lie on your back and simply rock back and forth.

For your review:

Did your baby like this exercise today?

_____

_____

How did you make it fun for both of you?

_____

_____

Did you need to modify anything?

_____

_____

Are you feeling stronger today?

_____

_____

TRANSITION:

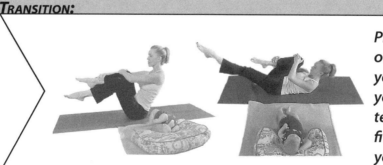

Place your left hand on your right knee and your right hand on your right ankle. Extend your left leg forty-five-degrees and roll your body to the floor.

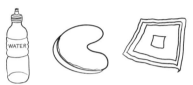

There are five exercises in this series; we will only do three.

GOAL: To strengthen your **powerhouse.**

POST-NATAL BENEFITS: This series targets and flattens those stubborn post pregnancy stomach muscles. Your baby will love tracking the movement of your arms and legs. You are like a human mobile!

What is needed:

NOTES:

Single Leg Stretch

△2 △3 △4 △5

POSITION:

LIE on your back with your head and shoulders curved off the ground. Your right leg is bent in to your chest with your right hand on your ankle and your left hand on your knee. Your left leg is extended at a forty-five-degree angle.

YOUR baby is in a bouncy chair or supportive pillow at your side about an arm's length away.

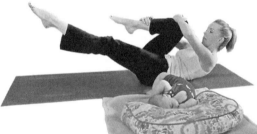

EXECUTION:

EXHALE as you pulse your right knee toward your chest two times, then switch legs and hands. Your left hand is on your left ankle, with your right hand on your left knee.

INHALE as you pulse your left leg in two times.

This is one set.

Do eight sets.

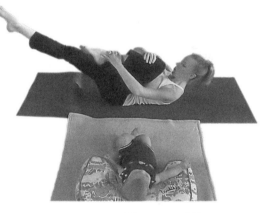

Helpful Hints:

Scoop your belly in and up.

Keep your neck and shoulders relaxed.

You can sustain one breath throughout the set (right and left) or breathe every time you switch legs.

MODIFICATION:

Take your extended leg up higher if you feel your lower back leave the floor or your stomach push out.

You can lower your neck and shoulders if you feel strain but only if you raised your legs to ninety-degrees.

For your review:
Did your baby like this exercise today?

_____

_____

How did you make it fun for both of you?

_____

_____

Did you need to modify anything?

_____

_____

Are you feeling stronger today?

_____

_____

TRANSITION:

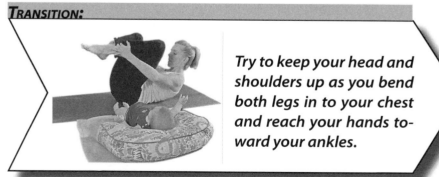

Try to keep your head and shoulders up as you bend both legs in to your chest and reach your hands toward your ankles.

What is needed:

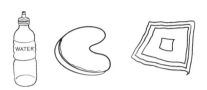

NOTES:

_____

_____

_____

_____

Double Leg Stretch

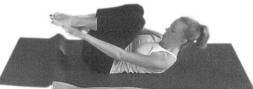

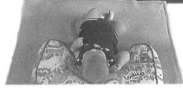

POSITION:

LIE on your back with your head and shoulders curled off the floor, knees bent. Your fingertips reach for your ankles.

EXECUTION:

INHALE as you extend your arms and your legs on the diagonal in opposite directions. Your legs should be turned out from the hip.

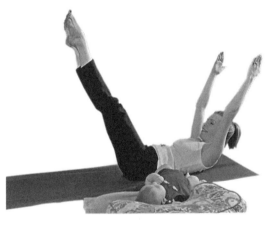

EXHALE as you parallel your legs and bend them back in while circling your arms around to your ankles.

This is one set.

Do four sets.

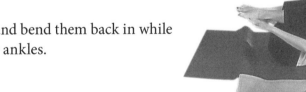

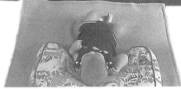

Helpful Hints:

It is very important that your back stay connected to the ground. **Imprint!**

*BABY CAN HOLD UP HER OWN HEAD AROUND **3–4** MONTHS.*

MODIFICATION:

If you feel strain in your back take your legs and arms directly to the ceiling—not on the diagonal.

 If you take your legs too low, you risk back strain—and you won't flatten your stomach muscles.

For your review:

Did your baby like this exercise today?

_____

_____

How did you make it fun for both of you?

_____

_____

Did you need to modify anything?

_____

_____

Are you feeling stronger today?

_____

_____

TRANSITION:

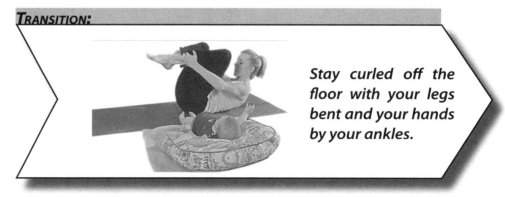

Stay curled off the floor with your legs bent and your hands by your ankles.

What is needed:

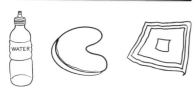

NOTES:

_____

_____

_____

_____

Helpful Hints:

Try to curl your chest up higher, rather than forcing your leg to your chest.

There should be a hollow space between your leg and chest.

Use your **powerhouse** to control your leg movements when switching legs.

Straight Leg Stretch

⚠ /1\ /2\ /3\ /4\ /5\

POSITION:

LIE on your back. Head and shoulders are still curled off the floor. Your belly is scooped in and up. Extend your right leg toward the ceiling and hold your ankle with both hands. Extend your left leg at forty-five-degrees or higher.

EXECUTION:

EXHALE and gently stretch your right leg in toward your upper body two times.

SWITCH legs:

GRAB your left ankle with both hands.

INHALE and gently stretch your left leg in toward your upper body two times. Keep your navel to spine and your upper back curled off the floor.

This is one set.

Do eight sets.

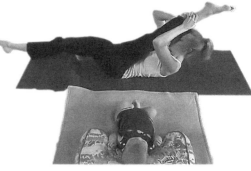

BLACK, WHITE AND RED WILL APPEAL THE MOST TO HER.

MODIFICATION:

If your **hamstrings** are tight, bend your leg or hold on to it at your calf (rather than your ankle) or at a higher point on your leg.

For your review:

Did your baby like this exercise today?

_____

_____

How did you make it fun for both of you?

_____

_____

Did you need to modify anything?

_____

_____

Are you feeling stronger today?

_____

_____

TRANSITION:

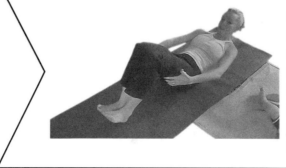

Bend both legs and lower your head and shoulders. Place your feet on the floor. Flex them and slide them away from your buttocks but keeping your legs bent. Place your hands behind your thighs and do one good ROLL UP.

Spine Stretch

What is needed:

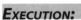

NOTES:

_____

_____

_____

_____

_____

GOAL: To articulate your spine and increase the space between each vertebra. This will help with your posture.

POST-NATAL BENEFITS: This exercise can relieve back ache associated with poor posture resulting from pregnancy and from holding your new baby all day.

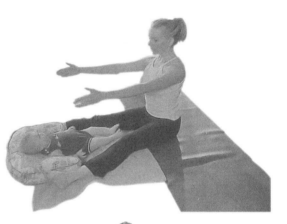

POSITION:

SIT tall with your lower legs on either side of your baby's pillow or chair. Your arms are extended in front of you, shoulder width apart and parallel to the floor palms facing in. Keep your shoulders reaching back and down in opposition.

EXECUTION:

INHALE to grow taller in your spine, lifting your ribs off your hips. Exhale as you round forward, starting with the top of your head. Keep your arms parallel to the floor. Reach the crown of your head toward your thighs.

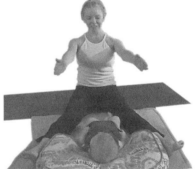

Helpful Hints:

Your feet and legs are relaxed.

Your head is the first to go and the last to arrive.

Your belly should feel like it goes up and under your **ribcage**.

Have fun with your baby. Gently shake your head from side to side or makes faces as you round over and up.

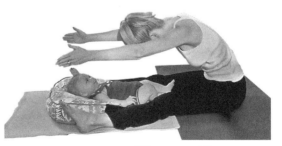

Pilates and Pregnancy

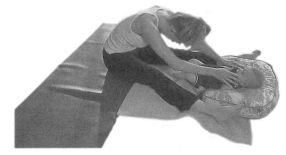

INHALE to start rolling up from the base of your spine. Exhale to completely uncurl by pulling your belly and ribs in toward your spine. Lower your arms to tickle your baby as you roll up. Return your arms to the starting position. Your head is the last to arrive.

This is one set.

Do six sets.

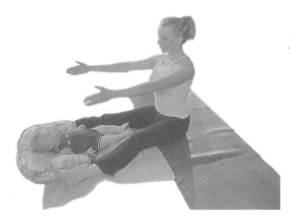

For your review:

Did your baby like this exercise today?

_____

_____

How did you make it fun for both of you?

_____

_____

Did you need to modify anything?

_____

_____

Are you feeling stronger today?

_____

_____

MODIFICATION:

If your **hamstrings** are tight, sit on a pillow or soften your knees.

You can keep your arms down the whole time if you feel strain in your neck and shoulders.

TRANSITION:

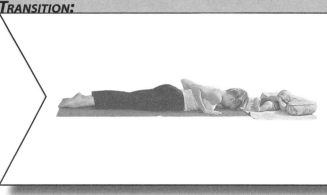

Move away from your baby and bring both legs together. Swing them around so that you are lying on your stomach with your head about four inches from your baby's feet.

Swan

What is needed:

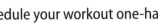

NOTES:

_____

_____

_____

_____

GOAL: To stretch your back.

POST-NATAL BENEFITS: This exercise can counteract the rounded shoulders and sunken chest that develop from holding and breast feeding your baby. What's better than a game of peek-a-boo that is also beneficial for your body?

POSITION:

LIE on your stomach with your legs reaching long, inner thighs together. Your pubic bone is tilted forward into the ground to help lengthen you lower back. Your hands are on the floor by your breasts. Keep your elbows close to your body.

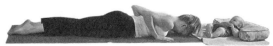

EXECUTION:

INHALE as you draw your belly and ribs in. Lengthen your torso off the floor. Exhale to lower down.

This is one set.

Do six sets.

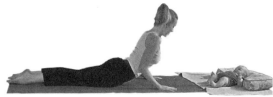

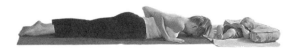

Helpful Hints:

Think of reaching your torso so long it has to curve up.

Keeping your arms slightly bent gives your **triceps** a great workout.

Support your back by pulling your belly in at all times.

Shoulders reach down your back.

Your focus is slightly down and in front of you, to keep the back of your neck long.

If breast tenderness is an issue, schedule your workout one-half hour after breast feeding.

For your review:

Did your baby like this exercise today?

_____

_____

How did you make it fun for both of you?

_____

_____

Did you need to modify anything?

_____

_____

Are you feeling stronger today?

_____

_____

MODIFICATION:

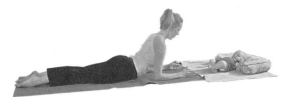

If you have hand and wrist problems, place your forearms on the floor and just think about reaching your torso long.

If you feel pain in your lower back, don't come up so high. Imagine you are in a slight **pelvic tilt.**

TRANSITION:

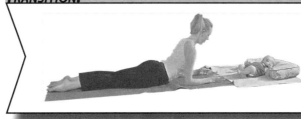

Come to your forearms with your shoulders down and your torso and neck long.

Single Leg Kick

What is needed:

GOAL: To stretch your **hip flexors** and **quadriceps**.

POST-NATAL BENEFITS: **SINGLE LEG KICK** can help relieve that tightness in the front of your legs and hips. Your baby can watch her favorite face—especially if your facial expressions are animated and playful.

NOTES:

POSITION:

LIE on your stomach, propped up on your forearms with your shoulders down. Your belly and ribs are pulled in. Your legs are reaching together and long, feet are pointed. Focus slightly down and about two feet in front of you to keep the back of your neck long.

EXECUTION:

EXHALE as you bend your right leg in a ninety-degree angle, flex and point your right foot at the top.

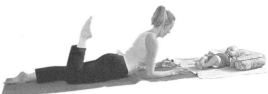

Helpful Hints:

Press into the floor with your forearms while pulling the bones of your arms backward from your shoulders. This will put your **scapulae** in the correct position.

Reach your knee away and your **hip bone** down so that you buttocks does not lift. This will allow a true stretch of your thigh and hip to occur.

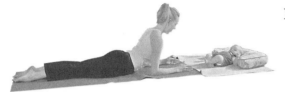

INHALE as you lower your right leg back down.

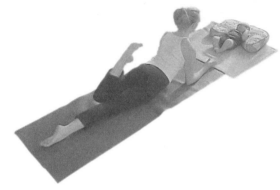

SWITCH legs:

BEND your left leg in with a pointed foot. Flex, then point your foot lower.

INHALE to lower.

This is one set.

Do five sets.

For your review:

Did your baby like this exercise today?

_____

_____

How did you make it fun for both of you?

_____

_____

Did you need to modify anything?

_____

_____

Are you feeling stronger today?

_____

_____

If you have knee problems, don't bend your knee past ninety-degrees.

TRANSITION:

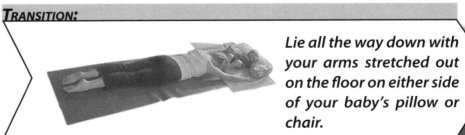

Lie all the way down with your arms stretched out on the floor on either side of your baby's pillow or chair.

Swimming

What is needed:

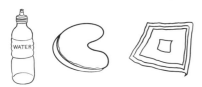

NOTES:

_____

_____

_____

Helpful Hints:

Keep your **powerhouse** active.

Stay in a slight pelvic tilt.

Reach from the back of your knee and heel to keep your leg straight.

Work in opposition so that you reach your fingers and toes away from your torso and your shoulders and hips toward your center.

GOAL: To strengthen your back muscles.

POST-NATAL BENEFITS: Back strength is as important as abdominal strength for healthy posture. This is a great exercise for anyone with back problems. Your baby will be able to track your hands as they rise and fall from her sight.

POSITION:

LIE on your stomach, legs together and long, feet pointed. Your forehead is on the floor and your pubic bone is gently pressing into the floor. Your arms are on the floor on either side of your baby.

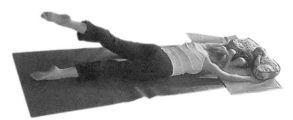

EXECUTION:

THERE ARE TWO PARTS TO THIS EXERCISE.
PART I IS A WARM UP.
PART II IS THE FULL SWIMMING EXERCISE.

EXECUTION: PART I:

KEEPING your forehead on the ground, inhale and reach your right arm so long it floats off the floor. Reach your shoulder down your back in opposition.

EXHALE as your arm lowers.

INHALE to raise your left arm. Exhale to lower.

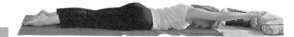

INHALE as you reach your right leg so long it floats off the floor. Keep your hip where it is. Exhale to lower your leg.

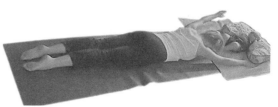

INHALE to reach your left leg so long it floats off the floor. Exhale as it lowers.

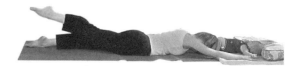

By 3 months she will love to play with others.

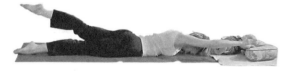

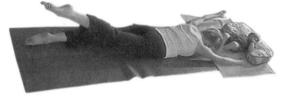

Inhale as you reach your right arm and left leg off the floor. Relax your neck and keep your forehead on the floor.

Exhale to lower.

Inhale to reach your left arm and right leg up.

Exhale to lower.

Execution: Part II:

Inhale both arms and legs and your head off the floor but keep your focus down.

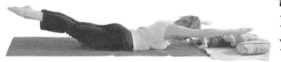

Alternate moving your opposite arm and leg up and down. Exhale for two counts; inhale for two counts.

That is one set.

Do Part II for four sets of two breaths per set.

Modification:

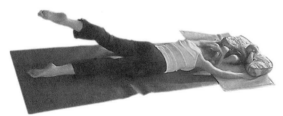

If you have shoulder problems, just work your legs.

For your review:
Did your baby like this exercise today?

_____

_____

How did you make it fun for both of you?

_____

_____

Did you need to modify anything?

_____

_____

Are you feeling stronger today?

_____

_____

Transition:

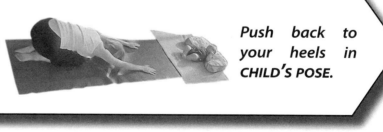

Push back to your heels in **Child's Pose.**

Child's Pose/A Little Piece of Heaven

What is needed:

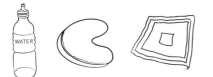

NOTES:

_____

_____

_____

_____

GOAL: To relax and stretch your back muscles.

POST-NATAL BENEFITS: Back strain isn't just from pregnancy. The weight of heavier breasts and the strain of carrying the baby often result in back pain among postpartum women. Babies need a break from stimulation, just like us. Allow him to enjoy these few seconds of stillness.

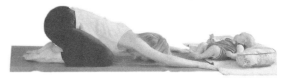

POSITION:

SIT on your feet with your heels together, toes apart. Your knees are **hip-width apart** with your arms back at your sides and your forehead on the floor.

EXECUTION:

PRACTICE your **BREATHING**. Try to release your back and neck muscles more with every exhale. Keep pulling your stomach off your thighs as you **ribcage** expands back and sideways on every inhale

Helpful Hints:

At this point you may have guessed that your **power-house** never fully disengages.

Try to stretch your back as you inhale.

BABIES BEGIN "BABBLING" AROUND 3 MONTHS.

MODIFICATION:

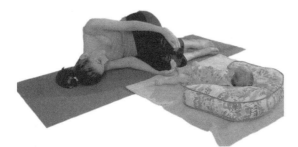

Place a pillow behind your knees or curl up on your side in a fetal position if you have knee pain.

For your review:

Did your baby like this exercise today?

_____

_____

How did you make it fun for both of you?

_____

_____

Did you need to modify anything?

_____

_____

Are you feeling stronger today?

_____

_____

TRANSITION:

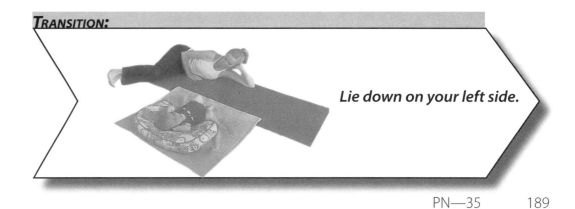

Lie down on your left side.

Side Kick Series

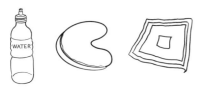

NOTES:

This is an entire series of exercises performed while lying on your side. We will do three in this series, first on the right and then on the left.

GOAL: To strengthen your **powerhouse** enabling your legs to stretch.

POST-NATAL BENEFITS: This series can elongate your body from head to toe while toning and stretching your legs and hips. Your baby will love looking at her human mobile and tracking your leg movements.

FRONT/BACK ⚠2 ⚠3 ⚠4 ⚠5

Helpful Hints:

When you kick front, imagine reaching your **tailbone** down and slightly back. To keep from arching as your leg goes back, imagine reaching your ribs down and your abdominal muscles up and in.

A smaller range of motion with no movement in your torso distortions will make you stronger and more flexible than simply letting your leg swing.

POSITION:

LIE on your left side with your left hand supporting your head. Your right hand is on the floor in front of your **sternum**. Reach both legs very long on the floor at a forty-five-degree angle from your torso. Keep your legs parallel, feet flexed. Try to create one line from your head to your tailbone by keeping your belly button to your spine and your **ribcage** down.

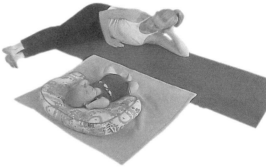

✱Your baby is on the supportive pillow or in the chair a leg's length or more in front of you.

INHALE to release your right leg off your left, hip-height.

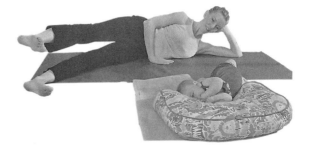

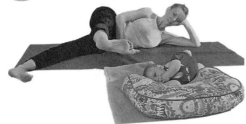

EXECUTION:

EXHALE and kick to the front with a double pulse without letting your leg move your torso in any way.

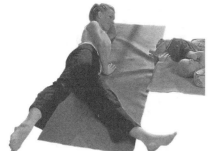

INHALE and point your right foot and reach your leg down and slightly behind you.

This is one set.

Do eight sets on the right.

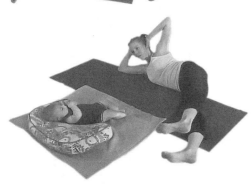

For your review:

Did your baby like this exercise today?

_____

_____

How did you make it fun for both of you?

_____

_____

Did you need to modify anything?

_____

_____

Are you feeling stronger today?

_____

_____

MODIFICATION:

Place your back against a wall if you cannot tell whether your torso is shifting.

ADVANCED: If you are very strong and your torso remains still, put both hands behind your head and prop yourself up on your left elbow, with your rib cage lifted.

TRANSITION:

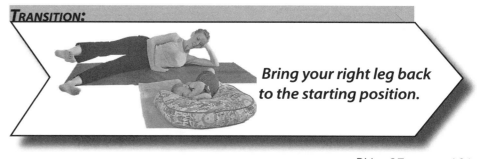

Bring your right leg back to the starting position.

Side Kick Series

What is needed:

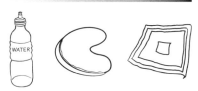

Notes:

_____

_____

_____

_____

_____

Up/Down

△1 △2 △3 △4 △5

POSITION:

WITHOUT rocking back in your hips, turn your right leg out and place your right heel on the instep of your left foot.

EXECUTION:

EXHALE, point your right foot, and release your right leg up to the ceiling.

INHALE, as you flex your foot and bring your leg back down.

This is one set set.

Do eight sets.

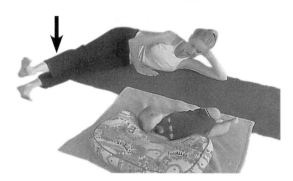

Helpful Hints:

Control your leg as it comes down.

Grow taller in your torso as your leg kicks up.

BABY DEVELOPS FULL COLOR VISION AROUND 6 MONTHS.

MODIFICATION:

Place your back against a wall to check whether you are shifting back.

ADVANCED: Place both hands behind your head as described earlier.

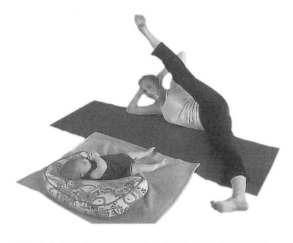

For your review:

Did your baby like this exercise today?

_____

_____

How did you make it fun for both of you?

_____

_____

Did you need to modify anything?

_____

_____

Are you feeling stronger today?

_____

_____

TRANSITION:

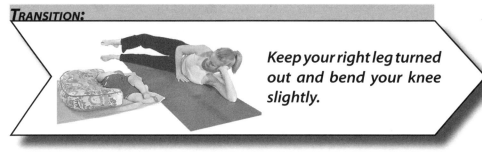

Keep your right leg turned out and bend your knee slightly.

What is needed:

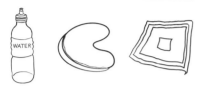

NOTES:

_____

_____

_____

_____

Helpful Hints:

Shake your leg before beginning to make sure your thigh muscle is relaxed.

The big muscle groups always want to take over. Real strength and length comes from balancing them with all the smaller, stabilizing muscles.

Small Circles

⚠1 ⚠2 ⚠3 ⚠4 ⚠5

POSITION:

BEND your right knee slightly and relax your foot. Your left leg is still straight and long with a flexed foot.

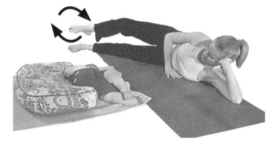

EXECUTION:

MAKE small circles from the top of your thigh. Relax your quadriceps muscle and initiate from your buttocks and **powerhouse**. Inhale for half the circle, exhale for half.

Do eight circles in one direction.

Pause and reverse the direction of the circle eight times.

MODIFICATION:

Place your back against a wall.

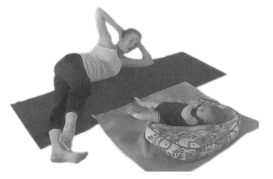

ADVANCED: Place both hands behind your head.

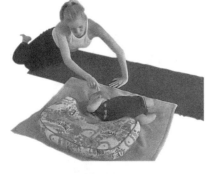

TRANSITION TO THE LEFT SIDE:

PUSH up to a seated position. Swing your legs around to the other side and lie down on your right side.

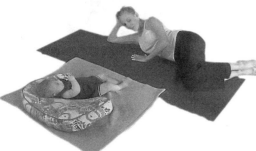

Repeat FRONT/BACK, UP/DOWN, AND SMALL CIRCLES *using your left leg.*

For your review:

Did your baby like this exercise today?

_____

_____

How did you make it fun for both of you?

_____

_____

Did you need to modify anything?

_____

_____

Are you feeling stronger today?

_____

_____

TRANSITION:

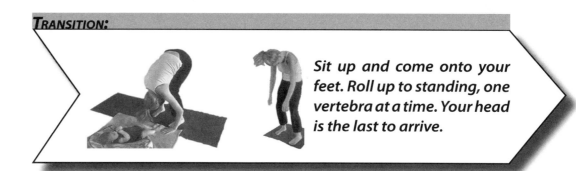

Sit up and come onto your feet. Roll up to standing, one vertebra at a time. Your head is the last to arrive.

Flat Back Punches/Pulling Weeds

What is needed:

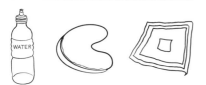

NOTES:

_____

_____

_____

_____

_____

Helpful Hints:

Try to keep your arms the exact height of your torso.

Stick your buttocks out slightly and wrap your abdominal muscles around to your back to achieve this flat back position.

GOAL: To strengthen your back and stretch your shoulders.

POST-NATAL BENEFITS: Hours of carrying your baby can leave your upper back and shoulders in a rounded position, this exercise helps target that area. Your baby gets to watch your face as you will be standing with your face directly over his.

POSITION:

COME close to your baby who is still in her supportive pillow. Your feet are parallel and **hip-width apart.** Soften your knees and bend forward from your hips. Your back will be as flat as a table top. Your focus is straight down at your baby. Bend your arms, your hands are in fists and keep your arms close to your torso.

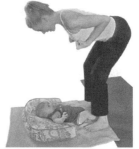

Flat Back Punches

EXECUTION:

INHALE and punch your right arm forward, palm down and your left arm back, palm up.

EXHALE and bend back.

SWITCH sides:

INHALE to punch your left arm forward and your right arm back.

EXHALE to bend back.

This is one set.

Do four sets

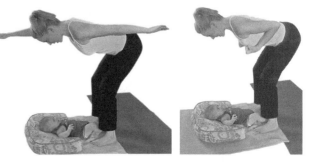

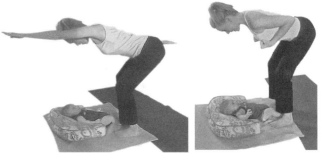

Pilates and Pregnancy

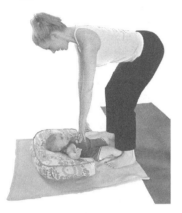

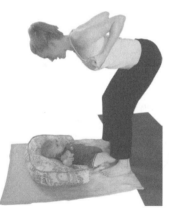

Pulling Weeds

EXECUTION:

WITHOUT rounding your back and shoulders, inhale to reach your arms straight down toward your baby. Wiggle your fingers then close your fist and pull your arms back to the starting position.

This is one set.

Do eight sets.

For your review:

Did your baby like this exercise today?

_____

_____

How did you make it fun for both of you?

_____

_____

Did you need to modify anything?

_____

_____

Are you feeling stronger today?

_____

_____

Helpful Hints:

Reach your shoulders back in opposition to your hands reaching down.

Make faces at your baby.

TRANSITION:

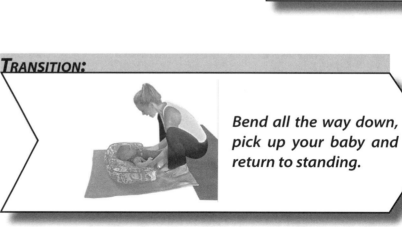

Bend all the way down, pick up your baby and return to standing.

Curls

What is needed:

NOTES:

_____

_____

_____

_____

Helpful Hints:

Only go as far as you can securely hold your baby.

Keep your focus forward for the shoulder press so as to not compress your lower back.

GOAL: To strengthen your chest, shoulders and arms.

POST-NATAL BENEFITS: Your baby is growing everyday. Why not use him as a weight so that your strength will match your needs? Your baby gets a little ride while playing peek-a-boo.

POSITION:

STAND with your legs parallel, **hip-width apart.** Keep your belly reaching in and up to prevent your back from arching.

HOLD your baby securely under her arm pits. Keep your upper arms glued to your torso.

EXECUTION:

Do four bicep curls.

INHALE as your arms lengthen so that his nose is in front of your **sternum.**

EXHALE as you bend your arms and bring his nose in front of your neck.

Do four shoulder presses.

INHALE to prepare, then exhale to lift your baby so that his navel is in line with your nose but no higher. Inhale to lower him down to the starting position.

Pilates and Pregnancy

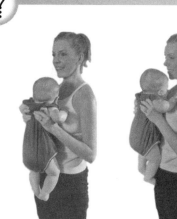

Do four chest presses.

EXHALE to prepare, then inhale to take your baby straight out from your chest *slightly*.

EXHALE to bring him back in.

RE-POSITION your baby to give his arm pits a break. Hug him, nuzzle him.

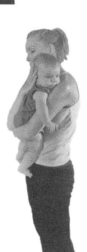

This is one set.

Do two sets of all three curls.

You can leave out any of the **CURLS** that are too difficult right now.

You may do these with weights if you don't feel completely comfortable doing them with your baby.

For your review:

Did your baby like this exercise today?

_____

_____

How did you make it fun for both of you?

_____

_____

Did you need to modify anything?

_____

_____

Are you feeling stronger today?

_____

_____

TRANSITION:

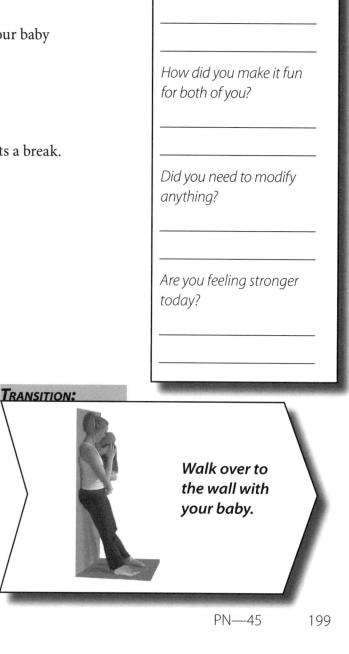

Walk over to the wall with your baby.

Squat

/1\ /2\ /3\ /4\ /5\

What is needed:

NOTES:

_____

_____

_____

_____

_____

Helpful Hints:

Your knees must be directly over your feet. Adjust your foot distance from the wall to achieve this.

Keep your **navel to spine** to support your torso.

GOAL: To strengthen your inner thighs, quadriceps and hamstrings.

POST-NATAL BENEFIT: A strong and toned lower body is essential in getting your body back to it's pre-pregnancy shape. Your baby will love being hugged close to your heart.

POSITION:

IMPRINT your back against the wall with your legs parallel, **hip-width apart.**

WALK your feet about six-to-eight inches away from the wall.

> It is very important that you are barefoot and standing on a non-slip surface.

EXECUTION:

WHILE securely holding your baby, inhale and slowly slide your back down the wall. Only go as far as you can while remaining strong and stable. Take a few breaths, then straighten your knees and slide back up the wall.

TALK to your baby, hug her and take a brief break.

This is one set.

Do two sets.

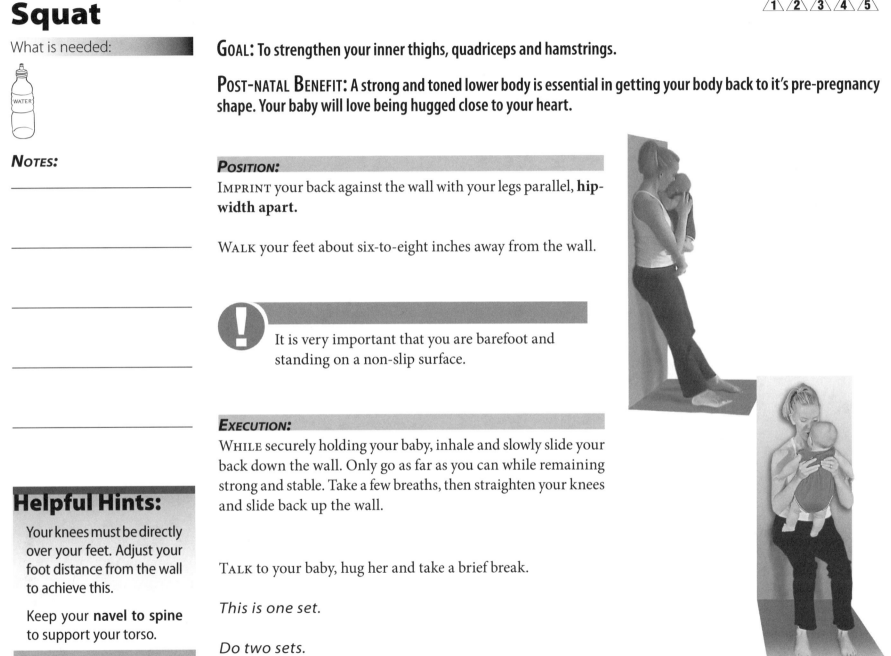

200   PN—46

Pilates and Pregnancy

YOUR BABY MAY IMITATE SOME FACIAL EXPRESSIONS AROUND 3-TO-4 MONTHS.

MODIFICATION:

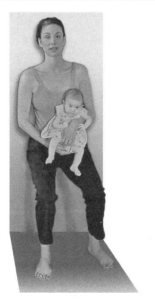

How you hold your baby is up to you and your baby. Just make sure she is safe and secure.

Come away from the wall and finish the exercise with your belly drawn in and your shoulders down and relaxed. Try to remember this feeling all day.

! If you feel at all tired or shaky, do not do this with your baby.

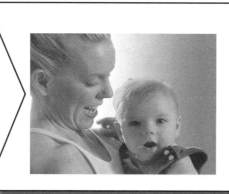

Thank your baby for being such a great workout partner!

HOW WAS YOUR DELIVERY? _____

1ST VISIT WITH YOUR OB/GYN? _____

WHAT WAS YOUR BABY'S WEIGHT AT BIRTH? _____

     AT 2 MONTHS? _____

     AT 3 MONTHS? _____

     AT 4 MONTHS? _____

     AT 5 MONTHS? _____

     AT 6 MONTHS? _____

HOW MANY DAYS PER WEEK DID YOU DO THIS PROGRAM? _____

WHAT EXERCISES FELT ESPECIALLY GOOD? _____

WHAT EXERCISES DID YOU AVOID? _____

HOW MANY DAYS A WEEK DID YOU WALK WITH YOUR BABY? _____

  HOW FAR? _____

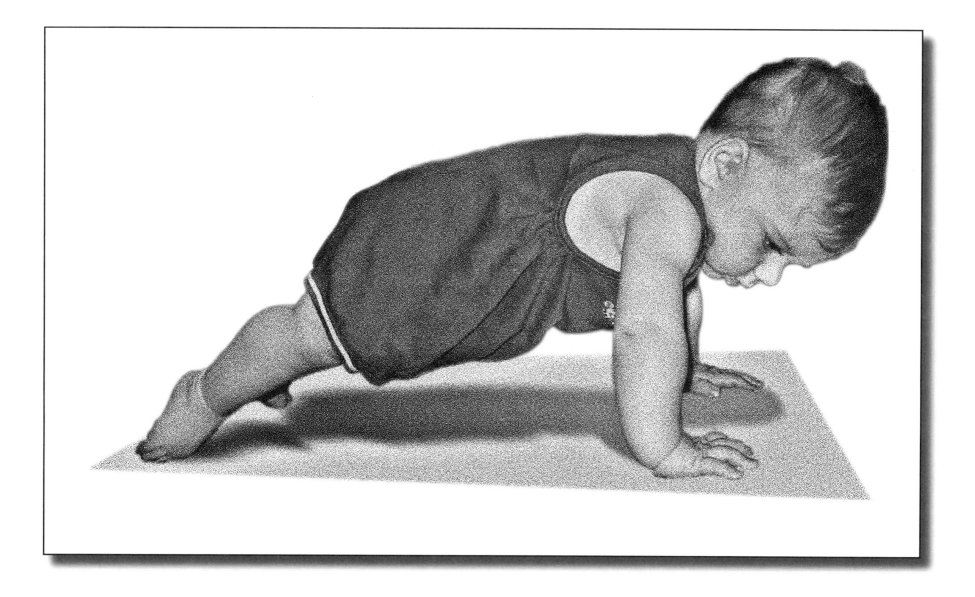

References

American College of Obstetricians and Gynecologists. *Planning Your Pregnancy and Birth*—3rd ed. Washington, DC: ACOG, 2000.

Sears, William, M.D. *The Pregnancy Book: A Month-by-Month Guide*. New York, NY: Little, Brown and Company, 1997.